Novel insights on
SGLT-2 Inhibitors

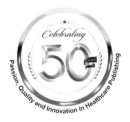

Novel Insights on
SGLT-2 Inhibitors

Authors

Rajeev Chawla

MD FRSSDI FACP (USA) FRCP (Edin) FACE (USA)

Senior Consultant Diabetologist and Director
North Delhi Diabetes Centre
New Delhi, India

Shalini Jaggi

Dip Diab (UK) Dip Endo (UK) FRSSDI FRCP (London, Glas, Edin) FACE (USA)

Consultant and Head
Department of Diabetology
Dr Mohans' Diabetes Specialities Centre
New Delhi, India

Foreword
Paresh Dandona

JAYPEE BROTHERS MEDICAL PUBLISHERS
The Health Sciences Publisher
New Delhi | London

Jaypee Brothers Medical Publishers (P) Ltd

Headquarters

Jaypee Brothers Medical Publishers (P) Ltd
4838/24, Ansari Road, Daryaganj
New Delhi 110 002, India
Phone: +91-11-43574357
Fax: +91-11-43574314
Email: jaypee@jaypeebrothers.com

Overseas Offices

J.P. Medical Ltd
83 Victoria Street, London
SW1H 0HW (UK)
Phone: +44 20 3170 8910
Fax: +44 (0)20 3008 6180
Email: info@jpmedpub.com

Website: www.jaypeebrothers.com
Website: www.jaypeedigital.com

Inquiries for bulk sales may be solicited at: jaypee@jaypeebrothers.com

Novel Insights on SGLT-2 Inhibitors / Rajeev Chawla, Shalini Jaggi

First Edition: **2020**

ISBN: 978-93-5270-680-8

Printed at: Samrat Offset Pvt. Ltd.

Foreword

We are in the golden era of innovation with respect to the discoveries in the field of diabetes over the past two decades. With the appropriate use of the drugs currently available, no patient with type 2 diabetes should remain uncontrolled and thus be vulnerable to diabetic complications. In this respect, three classes of drugs stand out: pioglitazone, a thiazolidenedione, and an insulin sensitizer, the glucagon like peptide-1 (GLP-1) receptor agonists and SGLT-2 inhibitors. All three have potent glucose lowering effects. However, it is remarkable that all have cardio-protective effects and may, therefore, potentially find use in prediabetic and non-diabetic populations. SGLT-2 inhibitors were launched into the market as glucose lowering agents exerting their action through the inhibition of glucose reabsorption at level of the proximal convoluted tubule in the kidney and the induction of glycosuria. Little did we realize that this action would be associated with other unique properties, including lowering of systolic blood pressure, cardioprotection and nephroprotection. The cardioprotective effect is the most marked in terms of cardiac failure. This action is so impressive that prospective clinical trials have been set up to assess this potential beneficial effect in non-diabetic populations. We still do not understand the mechanisms underlying these beneficial effects. Ketosis and ketonemia have been proposed as one mechanism leading to beneficial metabolic changes in the myocardium. However, further investigations and discoveries are still required to complete the mosaic related to the action of these drugs.

This book, edited by Drs Rajeev Chawla and Shalini Jaggi, provides an excellent opportunity for both the uninitiated and the specialist to learn about this class of drugs. I wish this book and the authors all the best wishes so that it can contribute to the translation of the golden age of innovation into a golden age of scientific and rational clinical practice.

Paresh Dandona MD PhD
SUNY Distinguished Professor
Head of Endocrinology, Diabetes and Metabolism
State University of New York and Kaleida Health
Director, Diabetes Endocrinology Center of Western New York

Preface

The scientific advancements over the last few decades have revolutionized the field of medicine, bringing in a much better understanding of the disease processes and their management. The growing epidemic of diabetes and obesity in current times pose a major challenge globally and is associated with a huge burden of comorbidities and complications. Last two decades have seen the advent of newer therapies, designer insulins as well as newer technologies and gadgets for management of diabetes, but unfortunately with the best of our efforts a vast majority of our patients are still not on optimum glycemic targets.

Type 2 diabetes is a progressive disease and there is always scope for newer agents that can address its multiple pathophysiological etiologies. One such class of new agents to be added to our armamentarium in recent times is the sodium-glucose transporter-2 inhibitors. These novel agents have changed the paradigm for diabetes management by inducing glycosuria in hyperglycemic patients to restore glycemia besides the added advantage of weight loss and reduction in BP. Hence, from being the conventional victim of hyperglycemia the kidney now has become a partner in the management of hyperglycemia. This book "Novel Insights on SGLT-2 Inhibitors" is an effort on our part to present to the readers an insight into how these agents came into being and have fast evolved today as potent antidiabetic drugs occupying the coveted place of preferred agents in all diabetes management algorithms globally owing to their efficacy, durability as well as pleiotropic benefits and cardiorenal protective effects. This book is a humble effort on our part to update the busy internists and primary physicians who because of their busy practices cannot find enough time to update themselves with the current concepts and placement as well as the future prospects of these new drugs in the management of diabetes. This book offers a crisp and balanced overview of all that we need to know about these agents not only for the beginners, but also for the established clinicians having a thirst for research and detail into this drug class. Every attempt has been made to highlight the clinically relevant points that serve as a quick referral guide on the topic concerned by means of a crisp introduction and conclusion encompassing each topic being discussed in the various chapters.

Rajeev Chawla
Shalini Jaggi

Acknowledgment

We have been associated on many platforms for the last few years and that is where we identified our common passion in writing which has finally brought us together in bringing out this first joint book. Each chapter is a joint effort—one prepared a skeleton and the other gave it shape and we tossed it to and fro multiple times, fine-tuning, layer by layer, till both of us were satisfied with the end result. In spite of our chronological differences in age, seniority and experience, the mutual respect and an eye for perfection that we share made this book eventually see light of the day in its current form.

It gives us extreme pleasure to express our gratitude to Mr Jitendar P Vij (Chairman), Jaypee Brothers Medical Publishers (P) Ltd, who not only prompted us to write this book, but also served as a catalyst throughout the project. Without his pursuance, it would not have been possible to write this book with our busy schedules. Himani Pandey, Development Editor, provided us the editorial support and helped us shape our writings into a concrete book. Their commitment and dedication to this endeavor is praiseworthy. We thank the publishers and the entire publication team for putting their tireless efforts to make this project possible.

We shall be failing in our duty if we don't acknowledge the contribution made by our families—spouses, parents and children in allowing us to take away precious hours from their kitty and spending them in researching and writing this book. Their support and good wishes along with their faith in us encouraged us to work together on this project.

We are equally grateful to all our patients who have provided us insights into diabetes and helped us master the practical tips in day-to-day management blessing us with such a vast clinical experience.

Contents

1
CHAPTER

The Evolution of SGLT-2 Inhibitors

INTRODUCTION

Diabetes mellitus is a state of chronic hyperglycemia secondary to multiple pathophysiological defects that include not only a dysfunction of the β-cells and α-cells resulting in impaired insulin and glucagon actions but also defective incretin axis, neurohormonal derangement in the brain as well as an increase in the glucose reabsorption in the kidneys. An understanding of these multiple etiological defects has stimulated researchers to search for novel agents targeting each of these mechanisms to optimize and individualize treatment of diabetes in current times. The latest agents to be added to our armamentarium are the sodium-glucose cotransporter-2 inhibitors (SGLT-2 inhibitors), commonly known as the gliflozins that primarily work by reducing the excessive renal glucose reabsorption that occurs in patients with diabetes. Following the discovery of phlorizin, the first natural SGLT-2 inhibitor, a number of synthetic glucoside analogs have been developed and are being used today while the search for newer agents is still ongoing. This chapter will introduce readers to the history and evolution of early-generation SGLT-2 inhibitors derived from natural plants leading to the development of the currently used prototypes of this class of agents and will give a glimpse into the recent advancement on the futuristic molecules in the pipeline.

THE FIRST NATURAL SGLT-2 INHIBITOR—PHLORIZIN AND ITS GLUCOSIDE ANALOGS

The first recognized natural substance with SGLT-2 inhibitory action was phlorizin, a dihydrochalcone compound isolated from barks of apple trees way back in 1835. Initially regarded as a treatment option for fevers, malaria and infectious diseases owing to its similarity with cinchona and willow tree extracts, the evolution of phlorizin as an inhibitor of renal glucose reabsorption that caused increase in urinary glucose excretion was reported almost five decades later by Chasis et al. The relationship between the glucose transport system of the proximal tubular brush border epithelium and phlorizin came to be established in 1970s. Several in vivo studies on diabetic animal models showed reduced fasting and/or postprandial blood glucose levels and increased insulin sensitivity following phlorizin administration. Katsuno et al. reported inhibition of both human SGLT-1 and SGLT-2 with phlorizin, with the inhibitory constant (Ki) values of 151 nM and 18.6 nM, respectively. In spite of its sufficient SGLT inhibitory actions, certain critical drawbacks disqualified phlorizin from further use as an antihyperglycemic agent. Most prominent of these was the low therapeutic selectivity of phlorizin for both SGLT-1 and SGLT-2. By inhibiting SGLT-1 primarily localized in the small intestine, phlorizin was shown to cause several gastrointestinal side effects, such as diarrhea, dehydration and malabsorption. Also, its absorption from small intestine was quite poor owing to its low oral bioavailability. Besides, phloretin, α-glycosidase catalyzed hydrolytic metabolite of phlorizin, strongly inhibits the ubiquitous glucose transporter 1 (GLUT1), which then may obstruct glucose uptake in various tissues.

These drawbacks lead to a quest for developing novel analogs of phlorizin that would have better stability, bioavailability, and higher selectivity for SGLT-2 receptors. Researchers then focused on the O-glucoside analogs of phlorizin eventually developing T-1095, an oral selective inhibitor of SGLT-2 that undergoes extensive hepatic metabolism into its active metabolite T-1095A. This metabolite demonstrated dose-dependent reduction in urinary glucose reabsorption with consequent reduction in blood glucose, triggering development of numerous other similar O-glucoside derivatives such as sergliflozin, remogliflozin and AVE2268 over the next few years. Though these agents minimized glucosidase-mediated degradation and increased systemic exposure, they were pharmacokinetically unstable and had incomplete pharmacological selectivity for SGLT-2. This eventually led to phasing out of these agents and shifted research toward other derivatives of phlorizin.

The first C-glucoside analogs of phlorizin were developed in 2000 which further lead to development of the currently used molecules—the first one being dapagliflozin, developed in 2008 by Meng et al. with lipophilic ethoxy substituents at position 4 on the B-ring of phlorizin as shown here in Figure 1. Dapagliflozin showed a dose-dependent glucosuric response and significantly reduced fasting and postprandial blood glucose levels as well as hemoglobin A1c (HbA1c) with significant weight loss and a 1,200-fold higher selectivity for human SGLT-2 versus SGLT-1 (IC50: 1.12 nM vs. 1,391 nM). Dapagliflozin was introduced and became commercially available first in Europe in 2012 followed by the United States Food and Drug Administration (USFDA) approval in January 2014 paving its way for use in US and eventually globally thereafter.

Canagliflozin, a thiophene derivative of C-glucoside was approved by the USFDA in 2013 with similar antihyperglycemic properties and an over 400-fold difference in selectivity for SGLT-2 versus SGLT-1 (IC50: 2.2 nM vs. 910 nM). The third gliflozin to hit

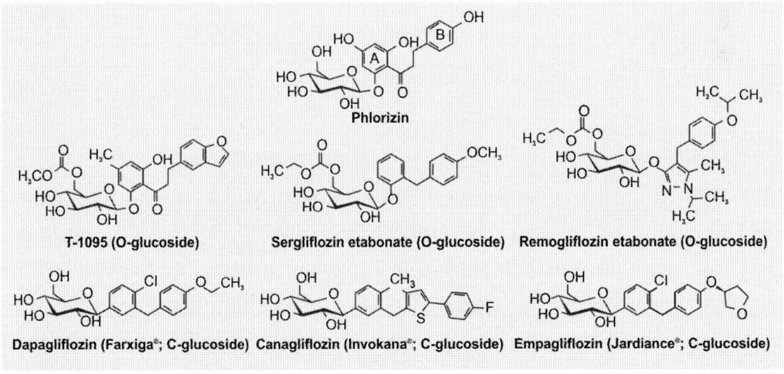

FIG. 1: Phlorizin and its major O- and C-glucoside analogs.

the global markets was empagliflozin characterized by the highest, i.e. 2,700-fold selectivity for SGLT-2 versus SGLT-1. Various other gliflozins such as ipragliflozin, tofogliflozin and luseogliflozin have since been developed, mainly by the Japanese, while others such as ertugliflozin and LX-4211 (sotagliflozin—a dual SGLT-2/SGLT-1 inhibitor) are also now the latest entrants into this arena.

SOPHORA FLAVESCENS (FABACEAE)

Sophora flavescens (S. flavescens) or the shrubby sophora is a popular Chinese shrub belonging to the pea family Fabacea. Its root, known as "Kushen", being rich in alkaloids and flavonoids, has traditionally been used for treating numerous diseases including dysentery, fever, jaundice, leukorrhea, scabies, pyogenic skin infections, swelling and also pain. Studies have also proven additional anti-inflammatory, antitumor, antianaphylactic, antiasthmatic, anti-microbial and immunoregulatory as well as cardiovascular protective effects. Research has further demonstrated that the methanol extract of this plant has a potent SGLT inhibitory activity. Three of these extracts, namely—(1) maackiain; (2) variabilin; and (3) formononetin, with isoflavonoid-based structures having a hydroxyl functional group, demonstrated exclusive SGLT-2 inhibitory activity. Also, flavanone compounds, the most potent being kurarinone and sophoraflavanone G, demonstrated extensive inhibition of both SGLT-2 and SGLT-1, with increased selectivity for SGLT-2 attributable to the common lavandulyl functional group at the C-8 position. Currently, SGLT-2 inhibitory effects of all nine isolated compounds of isoflavonoid glycosides from roots of S. flavescens have been demonstrated.

CONCLUSION

The identification of renal glucose reabsorption as an important pathophysiological contributor to hyperglycemia paved the way for SGLT-2 inhibition as a promising therapeutic strategy for treatment of type 2 diabetes mellitus. The last few years have shown the introduction of various SGLT-2 inhibitors derived from the natural active compound phlorizin, approved for use in type 2 diabetes both as monotherapy and as combination therapy with other antidiabetic agents including insulin. A number of these agents are now available globally while newer ones are being constantly developed and studied.

SUGGESTED READING

1. Abdul-Ghani MA, DeFronzo RA. Inhibition of renal glucose absorption: A novel strategy for achieving glucose control in type 2 diabetes mellitus. Endocr Pract. 2008;14(6):782-90.
2. Baynes JW. Role of oxidative stress in development of complications in diabetes. Diabetes. 1991;40(4):405-12.
3. Bays H. Sodium glucose co-transporter type 2 (SGLT2) inhibitors: Targeting the kidney to improve glycemic control in diabetes mellitus. Diabetes Ther. 2013;4(2):195-220.
4. Bickel M, Brummerhop H, Frick W, et al. Effects of AVE2268, a substituted glycopyranoside, on urinary glucose excretion and blood glucose in mice and rats. Arzneimittelforschung. 2008;58(11):574-80.
5. Chasis H, Jolliffe N, Smith HW. The action of phlorizin on the excretion of glucose, xylose, sucrose, creatinine and urea by man. J Clin Invest. 1933;12(6):1083-90.
6. Derdau V, Fey T, Atzrodt J. Synthesis of isotopically labelled SGLT inhibitors and their metabolites. Tetrahedron. 2010;66(7):1472-82.
7. Ehrenkranz JR, Lewis NG, Kahn CR, et al. Phlorizin: A review. Diabetes Metab Res Rev. 2005;21(1):31-8.
8. Gorboulev V, Schürmann A, Vallon V, et al. Na$^+$-D-glucose cotransporter SGLT1 is pivotal for intestinal glucose absorption and glucose-dependent incretin secretion. Diabetes. 2012;61(1):187-96.
9. Grempler R, Thomas L, Eckhardt M, et al. Empagliflozin, a novel selective sodium glucose cotransporter-2 (SGLT-2) inhibitor: Characterisation and comparison with other SGLT-2 inhibitors. Diabetes Obes Metab. 2012;14(1):83-90.
10. Han S, Hagan DL, Taylor JR, et al. Dapagliflozin, a selective SGLT2 inhibitor, improves glucose homeostasis in normal and diabetic rats. Diabetes. 2008;57(6):1723-9.
11. Hung HY, Qian K, Morris-Natschke SL, et al. Recent discovery of plant-derived anti-diabetic natural products. Nat Prod Rep. 2012;29(5):580-606.
12. Meng W, Ellsworth BA, Nirschl AA, et al. Discovery of dapagliflozin: A potent, selective renal sodium-dependent glucose cotransporter 2 (SGLT2) inhibitor for the treatment of type 2 diabetes. J Med Chem. 2008;51(5):1145-9.
13. Mudaliar S, Polidori D, Zambrowicz B, et al. Sodium-glucose cotransporter inhibitors: Effects on renal and intestinal glucose transport: From bench to bedside. Diabetes Care. 2015;38(12):2344-53.
14. Nomura S, Sakamaki S, Hongu M, et al. Discovery of canagliflozin, a novel C-glucoside with thiophene ring, as sodium-dependent glucose cotransporter 2 inhibitor for the treatment of type 2 diabetes mellitus. J Med Chem. 2010;53(17):6355-60.

15. Oku A, Ueta K, Arakawa K, et al. T-1095, an inhibitor of renal Na$^+$-glucose cotransporters, may provide a novel approach to treating diabetes. Diabetes. 1999;48(9):1794-800.

16. Rahmoune H, Thompson PW, Ward JM, et al. Glucose transporters in human renal proximal tubular cells isolated from the urine of patients with non-insulin-dependent diabetes. Diabetes. 2005;54(12):3427-34.

17. Rieg T, Masuda T, Gerasimova M, et al. Increase in SGLT1-mediated transport explains renal glucose reabsorption during genetic and pharmacological SGLT2 inhibition in euglycemia. Am J Physiol Renal Physiol. 2014;306(2):F188-93.

18. Rosenstock J, Aggarwal N, Polidori D, et al. Dose-ranging effects of canagliflozin, a sodium-glucose cotransporter 2 inhibitor, as add-on to metformin in subjects with type 2 diabetes. Diabetes Care. 2012;35(6):1232-8.

19. Rossetti L, Lauglin MR. Correction of hyperglycemia with phlorizin normalizes tissue sensitivity to insulin in diabetic rats. J Clin Invest. 1989;84(3):892-9.

20. Sato S1, Takeo J, Aoyama C, et al. Na+-glucose cotransporter (SGLT) inhibitory flavonoids from the roots of Sophoraflavescens. Bioorg Med Chem. 2007;15(10):3445-9.

21. Vallon V, Platt KA, Cunard R. SGLT2 mediates glucose reabsorption in the early proximal tubule. J Am Soc Nephrol. 2011;22(1):104-12.

22. Vallon V. The mechanisms and therapeutic potential of SGLT2 inhibitors in diabetes mellitus. Annu Rev Med. 2015;66:255-70.

23. Vestri S, Okamoto MM, de Freitas HS, et al. Changes in sodium or glucose filtration rate modulate expression of glucose transporters in renal proximal tubular cells of rat. J Membr Biol. 2001;182(2):105-12.

24. Vick H, Diedrich DF, Baumann K. Reevaluation of renal tubular glucose transport inhibition by phlorizinanalogs. Am J Physiol. 1973;224(3):552-7.

25. White JR. Apple trees to sodium glucose co-transporter inhibitors: a review of SGLT2 inhibition. Clin Diabetes. 2010;28(1):5-10.

26. Wright EM, Loo DD, Hirayama BA. Biology of human sodium glucose transporters. Physiol Rev. 2011;91(2):733-94.

Physiology of SGLT-2 Inhibition: Role of Kidneys in Glucose Homeostasis in Type 2 Diabetes Mellitus

INTRODUCTION

The role of kidneys in glucose homeostasis is now a well-known fact. The increase in glucose reabsorption from the renal tubules in a diabetic kidney contributes to worsening hyperglycemia. This understanding resulted in the development of novel agents, the sodium-glucose cotransporter-2 inhibitors (SGLT-2 inhibitors) that target this particular pathophysiological defect as an effective pharmacological strategy in treatment of type 2 diabetes mellitus (T2DM). To understand the pathology, we need to first focus on normal physiology of glucose homeostasis and the role of kidneys play in it. This chapter takes a look at the physiological role of kidneys in regulation of neoglucogenesis and glucose utilization, its pathophysiological impairment in T2DM, and reviews how these novel agents can effectively rectify this defect making them preferred oral agents for management of hyperglycemia in current times.

RENAL GLUCONEOGENESIS IN THE POSTABSORPTIVE STATE

In healthy individuals in the fasting or postabsorptive stage, the kidneys contribute about 20–25% of the glucose that is released into circulation via gluconeogenesis (15–55 g/day) while the liver releases the remaining glucose via both glycogenolysis and gluconeogenesis. Renal gluconeogenesis occurs primarily in the proximal tubular cells in the renal cortex and is regulated by insulin and catecholamines like adrenaline. Insulin reduces the release of glucose into circulation by directly inhibiting gluconeogenesis as well as by reducing availability of substrates such as glutamine, lactate and glutamate. On the other hand, adrenaline stimulates gluconeogenesis, increases supply of substrates, inhibits insulin secretion and reduces renal glucose uptake, and increasing the release of glucose into circulation.

In T2DM, the increased gluconeogenesis causes an increase in both renal as well as hepatic glucose release into circulation. The relative rise in renal gluconeogenesis has been documented to be significantly more than that in hepatic gluconeogenesis (300% vs. 30%). Also renal glycogenesis, which is minimal in healthy individuals, also contributes to the increased glucose release from kidneys in diabetes owing to glycogen accumulation in the diabetic kidney.

RENAL GLUCOSE RELEASE IN THE POSTPRANDIAL STATE

The postprandial state is marked by an increase in renal gluco-neogenesis than the postabsorptive state. Studies have demonstrated a greater than twofold increase in renal glucose release during the 4.5 hours postprandial period. This allows for repletion of the hepatic glycogen stores by suppressing hepatic glucose release. The increased endogenous glucose release in patients with T2DM increases the glucose output by roughly 30% (100 g vs. 70 g) as compared to healthy individuals. As insulin regulates renal glucose release, increasing insulin resistance reduces the suppression of renal glucose release. Thus, kidneys release increasing amounts of glucose in the postprandial state. An additional contributor to the increasing glucose is also an increase in renal glucose reabsorption that occurs due to the upregulation of renal glucose transporters (GLUTs) in this situation.

RENAL GLUCOSE TRANSPORT

Glucose conservation is an important function of the kidneys that filter 160–180 g of glucose daily in healthy individuals which is then reabsorbed within the proximal tubules. This reabsorption occurs through both SGLTs as well as GLUTs. The SGLT-mediated transport of glucose across the cell membrane occurs actively against its concentration gradient utilizing energy derived from the sodium electrochemical potential gradient (Fig. 1). This is maintained by the transport of intracellular sodium ions into blood through the sodium-potassium adenosine triphosphatase (Na$^+$/K$^+$-ATPase) pumps present in the basolateral membrane of the renal tubules. Binding of glucose to the GLUTs induces a conformational change potentiating the passive transport of glucose across the cell membrane from the intracellular space into the plasma.

The proximal renal tubule has two main subtypes each of the SGLT and GLUT transporters that are expressed at the luminal brush border and the basolateral membrane of the renal epithelium, respectively (Fig. 1). SGLT-2 is the high-capacity but low-affinity cotransporter which plays a major role in renal glucose reabsorption, coupling with the active transport of sodium and glucose in a 1:1 ratio in the early proximal tubule. This is then followed by reabsorption of glucose into circulation via the GLUT2. The remaining glucose is reabsorbed by SGLT-1, a high-affinity but low-capacity transporter within the distal part of the proximal tubule (sodium:glucose ratio of 2:1) and further reabsorbed into circulation through the GLUT1.

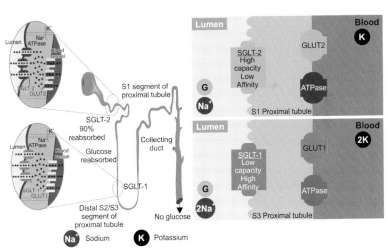

(ATPase: adenosine triphosphatase; GLUT2: glucose transporter 2; SGLT-2: sodium-glucose cotransporter-2)

FIG. 1: Glucose transport in tubular epithelial cells.

MECHANICS OF GLUCOSE REABSORPTION

- The electrochemical potential gradient existing across the brush border membrane provides the energy for active transport of glucose. It is driven by the sodium-potassium ATPase that pumps sodium out of the cell into blood while keeping the intracellular concentration low
- The SGLTs bind sodium followed by glucose. The sodium gradient sweeps both sodium and glucose from the lumen where sodium concentration is high, into the proximal tubular cells where sodium concentration is low because of the ongoing Na^+/K^+-ATPase pumping
- The glucose, thus, reabsorbed from the proximal tubule by the SGLT-2 is then released into blood by the GLUT2 while the GLUT1 releases glucose reabsorbed by SGLT-1.

The renal threshold for glucose excretion is increased in T2DM thus, causing an increase in glucose reabsorption. This increase in renal threshold for glucose excretion ensures that excess glucose is reabsorbed rather than excreted in urine. This pathophysiological increase in glucose reabsorption further aggravates the hyperglycemia, just contributing to the pathophysiology of T2DM.

The Figure 2 shows normal renal threshold for glucose excretion (RTG) and the right shift of RTG in T2DM.

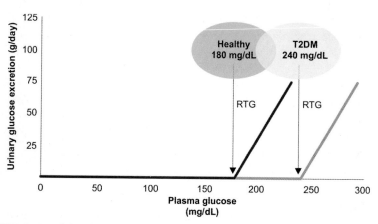

FIG. 2: Renal threshold for glucose excretion (RTG) is increased in type 2 diabetes mellitus (T2DM).

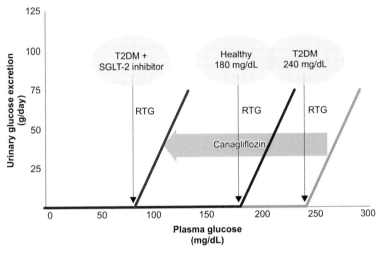

(SGLT-2: sodium-glucose cotransporter-2; T2DM: type 2 diabetes mellitus)

FIG. 3: SGLT-2 inhibitor lowers renal threshold for glucose excretion (RTG).

The Figure 3 depicts normal and diabetic RTG, with a far-left shift of RTG associated with SGLT-2 inhibition with an SGLT-2 inhibitor.

The SGLT-2 inhibitor blocks the SGLT-2 transporter, thus reducing the increased glucose reabsorption that was occurring due to hyperglycemia in T2DM. As a result, there is a re-setting of the hyperglycemia induced increased RTG back to normal levels, shifting the curve back, and in fact further far-left. This ensures that the excess glucose reabsorption is reduced and all the excess glucose can now be filtered out, inducing a glucosuria at reduced thresholds, thus correcting the hyperglycemia back to normal levels.

Above the saturation threshold, urinary glucose excretion increases in a linear fashion with increasing plasma glucose. The reabsorption curve is shifted to the right in T2DM.

GENETIC DEFECTS IN RENAL GLUCOSE TRANSPORT

Naturally occurring glycosuria has been shown to occur due to specific mutations in the *SGLT* genes. Glucose-galactose malabsorption (GGM), a rare disorder due to mutations in the SGLT-1, leads to malabsorption of these sugars because of a failure of the gastrointestinal epithelial cells to accumulate them across the brush border membrane. This manifests as diarrhea and dehydration in the neonatal period which can only be treated by omitting glucose and galactose (also transported by SGLT-1) from the diet. These subjects have only mild or absent glucosuria owing to the minor role of SGLT-1 in renal glucose reabsorption.

Familial renal glucosuria (FRG), a rare autosomal recessive disorder, results due to mutations in the *SLC5A2* gene that codes for SGLT-2. Heterozygous FRG is characterized by glucosuria of 0–10 g/day in the absence of renal tubular dysfunction even at normal plasma glucose concentrations. It is a benign condition and subjects are generally asymptomatic. Homozygous FRG, resulting in glucosuria to the tune of 200 g/day has rarely been described, though the available evidence from families with this condition indicates largely an asymptomatic presentation.

The learnings from the model of FRG clearly go on to show that glucosuria per se does not harm the kidneys in anyway. Hence the artificial glucosuria that is induced by using an SGLT-2 inhibitor to a patient with diabetes helps in correcting the pathophysiology and resets renal threshold for glucose excretion back to normal levels, and is purported to be absolutely harmless for the kidneys per se as in FRG which is a condition of natural glucosuria due to genetic defect.

CONCLUSION

Kidneys have an important role to play in regulation of glucose homeostasis through renal gluconeogenesis, glucose uptake and utilization and reabsorption of glucose from the proximal renal tubules. The RTG is defined as the plasma glucose concentration at which the capacity for glucose reabsorption is saturated and leads to glucosuria. It has been estimated to be around 180–200 mg/dL (10–11 mmol/L) in healthy individuals, and is seen to be increased in T2DM. As a result, the renal glucose reabsorbing capacity of the diabetic kidney increases, leading to worsening hyperglycemia. Inhibition of this excess glucose reabsorption and resulting glucosuria by inhibition of the SGLT-2 transporters in the proximal renal tubules by the SGLT-2 inhibitors corrects this pathophysiological defect and hence offers an efficacious and safe option for management of hyperglycemia in patients with T2DM.

SUGGESTED READING

1. Abdul-Ghani MA, Norton L, Defronzo RA. Role of sodium-glucose cotransporter 2 (SGLT 2) inhibitors in the treatment of type 2 diabetes. Endocr Rev. 2011;32(4): 515-31.

2. Bakris GL, Fonseca VA, Sharma K, et al. Renal sodium-glucose transport: role in diabetes mellitus and potential clinical implications. Kidney Int. 2009;75(12): 1272-7.

3. Bays H. From victim to ally: the kidney as an emerging target for the treatment of diabetes mellitus. Curr Med Res Opin. 2009;25(3):671-81.

4. Defronzo RA. Banting Lecture. From the triumvirate to the ominous octet: a new paradigm for the treatment of type 2 diabetes mellitus. Diabetes. 2009;58(4): 773-95.

5. Gerich JE, Meyer C, Woerle HJ, et al. Renal gluconeogenesis: its importance in human glucose homeostasis. Diabetes Care. 2001;24(2):382-91.

6. Gerich JE. Physiology of glucose homeostasis. Diabetes Obes Metab. 2000;2(6):345-50.

7. Gerich JE. Role of the kidney in normal glucose homeostasis and in the hyperglycaemia of diabetes mellitus: therapeutic implications. Diabet Med. 2010;27(2):136-42.

8. Shrayyef MZ, Gerich JE. Normal glucose homeostasis. In: Poretsky L (Ed). Principles of Diabetes Mellitus. New York: Springer; 2010. pp. 19-35.

9. Stumvoll M, Chintalapudi U, Perriello G, et al. Uptake and release of glucose by the human kidney. Postabsorptive rates and responses to epinephrine. J Clin Invest. 1995;96(5):2528-33.

10. Wright EM, Hirayama BA, Loo DF. Active sugar transport in health and disease. J Intern Med. 2007;261(1):32-43.

11. Wright EM. Renal Na(+)-glucose cotransporters. Am J Physiol Renal Physiol. 2001; 280(1):F10-8.

3

Beyond Glycosuria: Exploring the Intrarenal Effects of SGLT-2 Inhibition in Diabetes

INTRODUCTION

Sodium-glucose cotransporter-2 (SGLT-2) inhibitors are a novel class of oral antidiabetic drugs which produce renal glycosuria by inhibiting renal tubular glucose reabsorption via blocking SGLT-2 located at the luminal membrane of tubular cells of the proximal convoluted tubule. SGLT-2 inhibitors produce nephroprotection by not only improving glycemic control but also through glucose-independent direct renal effects and blood pressure-lowering. Glomerular hyperfiltration is likely to worsen diabetic nephropathy (DN). Glomerular hyperfiltration in diabetes occurs because of overactivation of renal tubular factors, including SGLT-2 and renin–angiotensin–aldosterone system. SGLT-2 inhibitors lead to reduction in hyperfiltration by inhibiting sodium reabsorption in the proximal tubule through tubuloglomerular feedback, causing afferent arteriole vasoconstriction and decrease fibrotic response of proximal tubular cells and inflammation. SGLT-2 inhibitors, however, do not produce significant glycemic reduction in patients with impaired renal function, given their mode of action. SGLT-2 inhibitors are in advantageous position as these function independent of β-cells, insulin secretion, and action. Therefore, their efficacy is maintained despite of progressive β-cell failure in type 2 diabetes mellitus (T2DM). They are very well tolerated, and carry a low risk of hypoglycemia.

The efficacy, safety, and mechanism of action of SGLT-2 inhibitors, in patients with normal and impaired renal function as mild, moderate, or severe renal impairment, is discussed. Beneficial effects of SGLT-2 inhibitors on renal function especially on albuminuria, hyperfiltration, and diabetic tubulointerstitial fibrosis are also discussed here.

SGLT-MEDIATED GLUCOSE TRANSPORTATION

Although glucose is the main fuel and source of energy but sustained hyperglycemia is driver of diabetic complications. Glucose is retained through number of biochemical processes and complicated transport systems. Kidneys try to preserve glucose via tubular glucose reabsorption through sodium-glucose cotransporters (SGLTs), secondary active cotransporters, and facilitative glucose transporters (GLUTs). SGLT-1 and SGLT-2, which are located in the brush border of the tubular cells at the proximal tubule, are members of the *SLC5* gene family and are secondary active SGLTs. SGLT-2 cotransporters have low affinity but very high capacity for glucose transportation and 1:1 sodium-glucose coupling and reabsorb approximately 80–90% of the filtered glucose. SGLT-1 transporters are located in the straight (S3) segment of the proximal tubule and have high affinity/low capacity for glucose and 2:1 sodium-glucose coupling and reabsorb the remaining 10–20% of glucose that "escapes" SGLT-2 reabsorption. SGLT-1 transporters are mainly expressed in the enterocytes of the small intestine apart from the kidney and facilitate both galactose and glucose absorption.

FACILITATIVE GLUCOSE TRANSPORTERS

Glucose transporter 1 and GLUT2 are part of GLUT (SLC2A) protein family and function as facilitative glucose transporters. GLUT1 facilitates glucose diffusion from the tubular cells intracellular space to the renal interstitial through the basolateral membrane at the proximal straight tubule (S3 segment) and GLUT2 at proximal convoluted (S1/2 segment) tubule.

MECHANISM OF TUBULAR GLUCOSE REABSORPTION (FIG. 1)

Sodium-potassium adenosine triphosphate (ATP)ase is located in the basolateral membrane of proximal tubular cells (PTCs) and is an active transporter and constitutes the source of energy for the glucose reabsorption transport system. Main fuel for the transportation of sodium ions to the kidney interstitium through the basolateral membrane of tubular cells comes from ATP hydrolysis. A negative electrical potential is created due to reduction of the intracellular sodium concentration which then induces sodium diffusion from the tubular lumen to the tubular intracellular space through SGLT cotransporters simultaneously driving glucose against its gradient, from the lumen into the tubular cells. Glucose diffuses to the kidney interstitium through GLUTs at the basolateral membrane after entering the tubular cells.

The sodium-potassium ATPase pump a primary active counter-transporter, is located at the tubular cells of the S1 and S3 segment of the proximal convoluted tubule. It exports sodium to the interstitium and imports potassium. Required energy for this function comes

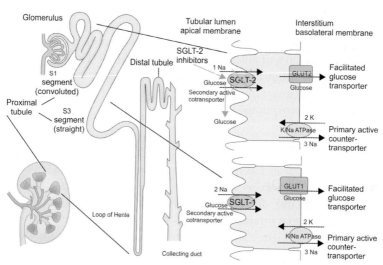

(GLUT2: glucose transporter 2; SGLT-2: sodium-glucose cotransporter-2)

FIG. 1: A model for renal glucose reabsorption.

from ATP-ADP transformation while sodium gradient needed for the operation comes from this pump. Sodium transportation happens along its gradient while glucose moves against its electrochemical gradient. GLUTs located at the basolateral membrane of the tubular cells facilitate passive glucose diffusion intracellularly to the interstitium. Concerning SGLTs, cotransporters on the brush border of tubular cells, SGLT-2 is located at the S1 segment and has 1:1 sodium to glucose stoichiometry while SGLT-1 is found at the S3 segment and has 2:1 stoichiometry.

PHYSIOLOGY OF GLUCOSE REABSORPTION

Kidneys filter 160–180 g of glucose daily in healthy individuals which is then reabsorbed within the proximal tubules leading to glucose conservation. Glucose filtered by the glomerular capillary membrane passes into the tubular lumen. Under normoglycemic conditions, the blood glucose concentration is 90–100 mg/dL and glomerular filtration rate (GFR) is about 180 per day. Approximately 162–180 g of glucose filters from the Bowman's capsule into the tubular lumen which is reabsorbed by the tubular GLUTs; hence, in a nondiabetic person, glucose is not excreted in the urine. With increasing hyperglycemia, tubular glucose reabsorption increases linearly till SGLTs reach their maximum transport capacity leading to saturation of glucose transport system. Transport maximum (TmG) corresponds with a blood glucose level of approximately 300 mg/dL, referred as the threshold for glucose (300 mg/dL is the quotient of TmG 375 mg/min and GFR 125 mL/min) and for the glucose tubular transport system in adults, it is about 375 mg/min. Once glucose level is above the level of TmG, excess glucose filtered is not reabsorbed and passes into urine.

ALTERATIONS OF RENAL GLUCOSE REABSORPTION IN DIABETES

Above the saturation threshold, with increasing plasma glucose, urinary glucose excretion increases in a linear fashion. The reabsorption curve gets shifted to the right in T2DM. TmG is 20% elevated in diabetics compared with healthy adults. In hyperglycemic states, glucose reabsorption is enhanced and hyperglycemia is further exacerbated because the mechanism of energy retention through glucose reabsorption becomes maladaptive in diabetic patients.

GENETIC DEFECTS IN RENAL GLUCOSE TRANSPORT

Renal glycosuria has been shown to occur due to specific mutations in the *SGLT* genes. Glucose-galactose malabsorption (GGM), a rare disorder due to mutations in the SGLT-1, leads to malabsorption of these sugars because of failure of the gastrointestinal epithelial cells to accumulate them across the brush border membrane. This manifests as diarrhea and dehydration in the neonatal period which improves by omitting glucose and galactose (also transported by SGLT-1) from the diet. These subjects have either mild or no glucosuria owing to the minor role of SGLT-1 in renal glucose reabsorption.

Familial renal glucosuria (FRG), a rare autosomal recessive disorder, results due to mutations in the *SLC5A2* gene that code for SGLT-2. Heterozygous FRG is a benign condition and does not have any renal tubular dysfunction but leads to glucosuria of 0–10 g/day even at normal plasma glucose concentrations. Homozygous FRG, with glucosuria of 200 g/day is rarely seen though this condition is largely asymptomatic. Encouraging initial studies on SGLT-2 inhibitors along with benign features of FRG stimulated further research into SGLT-2 inhibition as a therapeutic intervention for T2DM.

SGLT-2 INHIBITORS OFFER RENOPROTECTION

Sodium-glucose cotransporter-2 inhibitors not only improve glycemia but offer renoprotection through nonglycemic benefits in type 2 diabetics. Various studies have shown that glucose entry into tubular cells results into tubulointerstitial fibrosis, involving both PTCs, basement membrane alterations, and interstitial fibrosis leading to development of diabetic nephropathy. More evidence is emerging that SGLT-2 inhibitors, having beneficial effects on the afferent renal arteriole (constriction of the afferent arteriole), once combined with renin–angiotensin–aldosterone system (RAAS) inhibition which induces changes in R_E (efferent arteriole vasodilatation), may have cumulative renoprotective effect.

CONCLUSION

Kidneys till date have been victim of hyperglycemia but presently are being used as a partner in management of T2D. SGLT-2 inhibitors, a new class of antihyperglycemic agent, induce significant glucosuria and reduce hemoglobin A1c (HbA1c) and fasting plasma glucose (FPG) levels. SGLT-2 inhibitors work independent of β-cells and do not interfere with insulin secretion and action; hence, β-cell progressive failure does not impair their efficacy. Efficacy of these agent decreases with stages of renal impairment; however, as the glucosuric effect depends on renal function. SGLT-2 inhibition results in weight and blood pressure reduction due to consistent calorie loss and osmotic diuresis as a result of glucosuria. SGLT-2 inhibitors are generally well tolerated with very low risk of hypoglycemia and the most common adverse events being urinary tract infections (UTIs) and gastrointestinal disorders(GIs) but these can be minimized by ensuring enough oral liquids intake and maintaining personal hygiene.

SUGGESTED READING

1. Abdul-Ghani M, DeFronzo R. Inhibition of renal glucose reabsorption: a novel strategy for achieving glucose control in type 2 diabetes mellitus. Endocr Pract. 2008;14:782-90.
2. Abdul-Ghani M, DeFronzo R. Lowering plasma glucose concentration by inhibiting renal sodium-glucose co-transport. J Intern Med. 2014;276:352-63.
3. Berhan A, Barker A. Sodium glucose co-transport 2 inhibitors in the treatment of type 2 diabetes mellitus: a meta-analysis of randomized double-blind controlled trials. BMC Endocr Disord. 2013;13:58.
4. DeFronzo R, Davidson J, Del Prato S. The role of the kidneys in glucose homeostasis: a new path towards normalizing glycaemia. Diabetes Obes Metab. 2012;14:5-14.
5. DeFronzo R. From the triumvirate to the ominous octet: a new paradigm for the treatment of type 2 diabetes mellitus. Diabetes. 2009;58:273-95.
6. Ferrannini E, Veltkamp S, Smulders R, et al. Impact of chronic kidney disease and sodium-glucose cotransporter 2 inhibition in patients with type 2 diabetes. Diabetes Care. 2013;36:1260-5.
7. Gilbert R, Cooper M. The tubulointerstitium in progressive diabetic kidney disease: more than an aftermath of glomerular injury? Kidney Int. 1999;56:1627-37.

8. Hediger M, Rhoads D. Molecular physiology of sodium-glucose cotransporters. Physiol Rev. 1994;74:993-1026.
9. Jerums G, Premaratne E, Panagiotopoulos S, et al. The clinical significance of hyperfiltration in diabetes. Diabetologia. 2010;53:2093-104.
10. Magee G, Bilous R, Cardwell C, et al. Is hyperfiltration associated with the future risk of developing diabetic nephropathy? A meta-analysis. Diabetologia. 2009;52:691-7.
11. Novikov A, Vallon V. Sodium glucose cotransporter 2 inhibition in the diabetic kidney: an update. Curr Opin Nephrol Hypertens. 2015;24:1-9.
12. Ruggenenti P, Porrini E, Gaspari F, et al. Glomerular hyperfiltration and renal disease progression in type 2 diabetes. Diabetes Care. 2012;35:2061-8.

4

Cardiovascular Outcome Trials with SGLT-2 Inhibitors

INTRODUCTION

Diabetes and cardiovascular disease (CVD) go hand in hand and it was not till very long ago that diabetes was considered a CVD risk equivalent. Atherosclerotic CVD is considered the most prevalent cause of mortality and morbidity in patients with diabetes the world over, across both genders. Besides diabetes, common risk factors for CVD include hypertension and dyslipidemia, and most often all are seen to coexist. There is sufficient evidence to indicate that optimum control of each of these risk factors independently has a role in reducing risk of developing CVD. The management of type 2 diabetes mellitus (T2DM) has shifted from being glucocentric to a more comprehensive strategy that aims to reduce cardiovascular (CV) morbidity and mortality. In the last few years, a number of CV outcome trials with the newer antidiabetes drugs like dipeptidyl peptidase-4 (DPP-4) inhibitors, glucagon-like peptide-1 (GLP-1) receptor agonists, and sodium-glucose cotransporter-2 (SGLT-2) inhibitors have proven the CV safety of these drugs.

The three recently completed landmark CV outcome trials with SGLT-2 inhibitors have not only established the CV safety of these drugs, but have changed the treatment paradigms for T2DM management by demonstrating unprecedented cardiorenal benefits. The CV outcome trial with empagliflozin named the Empagliflozin Cardiovascular Outcome Event Trial in Type 2 Diabetes Mellitus Patients (EMPA-REG OUTCOME) trial proved superiority of empagliflozin in reducing CV outcomes and all-cause mortality in T2DM patients with established atherosclerotic cardiovascular disease (ASCVD). This was followed by the Canagliflozin Cardiovascular Assessment Study (CANVAS) Program where canagliflozin proved to be superior in CV outcome but not CV or all-cause mortality. Another interesting observation was a 1.97-fold higher incidence of low extremity amputation with canagliflozin treatment. Further to this, a recent analysis with the USA Food and Drug Administration (FDA) Adverse Event Reporting System demonstrated significantly higher frequency of amputation with canagliflozin compared with non-SGLT-2 inhibitors [proportional reporting ratio (PRR) of 5.33 (95% confidence interval (CI) 4.04–7.04)], which was also higher than other SGLT-2 inhibitors; the PRR for dapagliflozin was 0.25 (95% CI 0.03–1.76), and for empagliflozin it was 2.37 (95% CI 0.99–5.70). So far, there is no clear explanation for this disturbing result. However, findings from the OBSERVE-4D trial—In a real-world analysis of more than 700,000 patients with T2DM, adults with T2DM with and without established CVD treated with the canagliflozin did not have an increased risk for below-the-knee amputation compared with patients assigned SGLT-2 inhibitors or other antidiabetes therapies. Most recently, in DECLARE-TIMI 58 with its two primary efficacy analyses, dapagliflozin did not result in a lower rate of major adverse cardiovascular event (MACE) but did result in a lower rate of CV death or hospitalization for heart failure (HHF) as co-primary endpoint. Various hypothesis including metabolic and hemodynamic mechanisms have been proposed to explain for these results, though the exact mechanistic explanations are yet awaited.

A number of questions arise regarding the reduction in CV outcomes trials with SGLT-2 inhibitors. First, the extent to which the trials are relevant to only the population included in the trial is unclear. Second, are the CV benefits observed in these trials driven by, or at least partially explained by, a reduction in hyperglycemia or other mechanisms? Third, is this a drug class effect or does it differ between individual SGLT-2 inhibitors? Therefore, it is crucial to interpret these results of recent trials with SGLT-2 inhibitors correctly.

CARDIOVASCULAR OUTCOME TRIALS WITH SGLT-2 INHIBITORS (FLOWCHART 1)

Empagliflozin Cardiovascular Outcome Event Trial in Type 2 Diabetes Mellitus Patients Trial with Empagliflozin

In the EMPA-REG OUTCOME trial, 7,020 patients with long-standing T2DM (>10 years in 57% of the patients) with a mean age of 63 years at high risk of CVDs with >99% patients having established CVD [76% had coronary artery disease, 47% had history of myocardial infarction (MI)], were randomly assigned into three groups (placebo, empagliflozin 10 mg/day and empagliflozin 25 mg/day) and were followed for a median of 3.1 years. Mean baseline hemoglobin A1c (HbA1c) was 8.1%. Background diabetes treatment was first unchanged for 12 weeks. Placebo-adjusted mean reductions in

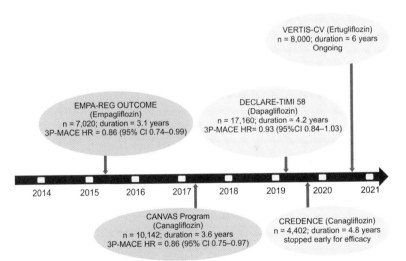

(CANVAS: Canagliflozin Cardiovascular Assessment Study; CI: confidence interval; DECLARE-TIMI 58: Dapagliflozin Effect on Cardiovascular Events-Thrombolysis in Myocardial Infarction 58; EMPA-REG OUTCOME: Empagliflozin Cardiovascular Outcome Event Trial in Type 2 Diabetes Mellitus Patients; HR: hazard ratio; SGLT-2: sodium-glucose cotransporter-2)

FLOWCHART 1: EMPA-REG, CANVAS, DECLARE-TIMI program and CREDENCE are complete and published.

HbA1c in the empagliflozin treatment groups were −0.54% at 12 weeks and −0.24% at 206 weeks. The primary endpoints defined as three-point major adverse CV events (3P-MACE) included death from CV causes, nonfatal MI and nonfatal stroke. The trial showed a primary composite of 3P-MACE reduction by 14% (p <0.001 for noninferiority; p = 0.04 for superiority). With no significant reduction in the relative risk of stroke or MI, this MACE risk reduction was primarily driven by a 38% relative risk reduction in CV death [hazard ratio (HR), 0.62; 95% CI, 0.49–0.77; p <0.001]. Furthermore, there was a 32% relative risk reduction in all-cause mortality (HR, 0.68; 95% CI, 0.57–0.82; p <0.001) and a 35% relative risk reduction in the incidence of HHF (HR, 0.65; 95% CI, 0.50–0.85; p = 0.002).

Canagliflozin Cardiovascular Assessment Study Program with Canagliflozin (Fig. 1)

This study program integrated data from two trials involving a total of 10,142 participants with T2DM and either established CVD or those at high CV risk. The mean age of the participants was 63.3 years, 35.8% were women, the mean duration of diabetes was

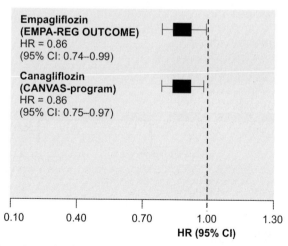

(CI: confidence interval; EMPA-REG OUTCOME: Empagliflozin Cardiovascular Outcome Event Trial in Type 2 Diabetes Mellitus Patients; HR: hazard ratio)

FIG. 1: EMPA-REG OUTCOME trial with empagliflozin and Canagliflozin Cardiovascular Assessment Study (CANVAS) program.

13.5 years and 65.6% had an established history of CVD. Participants in each trial were randomly assigned to receive canagliflozin 100 mg or 300 mg daily or placebo and were followed for a mean of 188.2 weeks. The primary outcome was a composite of death from CV causes, nonfatal MI, or nonfatal stroke. The rate of the primary outcome was lower with canagliflozin than with placebo (occurring in 26.9 participants vs. 31.5 participants per 1,000 patient-years; HR, 0.86; 95% CI, 0.75–0.97; p <0.001 for noninferiority; p = 0.02 for superiority). Approximately, 34% of the cohort was enrolled for primary prevention (age ≥50 years, no known coronary artery disease/CVD/peripheral artery disease, at least two risk factors). Higher event rates were observed in the secondary prevention subset. Canagliflozin in comparison to placebo, reduced the primary endpoint (p for interaction = 0.18), heart failure hospitalization (p for interaction = 0.91), and progression to albuminuria (p for interaction = 0.48) in both subgroups. In both subgroups, canagliflozin was associated with increased incidence of lower extremity amputations (p for interaction = 0.63).

Real-world Data with Canagliflozin, Dapagliflozin and Empagliflozin—CVD-REAL 1 Study

The CVD-REAL 1 study looked at the effects of the three SGLT-2 inhibitors versus other glucose-lowering drug classes on HHF and death in real-world practice. The researchers compared data from 309,056 patients newly initiated on either SGLT-2 inhibitors or other glucose-lowering drugs (oGLD) from six countries including the USA, UK, Norway, Denmark, Sweden and Germany. It was observed that after propensity matching, SGLT-2 inhibitors were significantly associated with lower rates of HHF (HR = 0.61; 95% CI, 0.51–0.73) and death (HR = 0.49; 95% CI, 0.41–0.57). Since CANVAS program also had positive outcomes for HHF as shown in EMPA-REG as well, this cohort study supported the two clinical trial results as being a class effect.

CVD-REAL 2 Study

As the population evaluated in CVD-REAL 1 was predominantly Caucasian, it was necessary to validate that SGLT-2 inhibitors as a class had similar effects in Asian and other population as well.

Therefore, CVD-REAL 2, a real-world study, was done. The study examined a broad range of CV outcomes in >400,000 type 2 diabetic patients on SGLT-2 inhibitors or oGLD across six countries in Asia Pacific, Middle East and North America. New patients on SGLT-2 inhibitors and oGLD were identified via claims, medical records and national registries in South Korea, Japan, Singapore, Israel, Australia and Canada. HRs for death, HHF, death or HHF, MI and stroke were assessed by country and pooled using weighted meta-analysis.

In the SGLT-2 inhibitors group, patients on dapagliflozin, empagliflozin, ipragliflozin, canagliflozin, tofogliflozin and luseo-gliflozin were included and accounted for 75%, 9%, 8%, 4%, 3% and 1% of exposure time, respectively. In all, there were 235,064 episodes of treatment initiation in each group after propensity-matching; about 27% of the patients had established CVD. Patient characteristics were well-balanced between groups. It was observed that the use of SGLT-2 inhibitors was associated with lower risk of death (HR, 0.51; 95% CI, 0.37–0.70; p <0.001), HHF (HR, 0.64; 95% CI, 0.50–0.82; p = 0.001), death or HHF (HR, 0.60; 95% CI, 0.47–0.76; p <0.001), MI (HR, 0.81; 95% CI, 0.74–0.88; p <0.001) and stroke (HR, 0.68; 95% CI, 0.55–0.84; p <0.001) versus other oGLD. A consistency in results was observed across all the countries in different ethnic populations and across different patient subgroups including those with and without pre-established ASCVD demonstrating a lower risk of CV events in patients initiated on SGLT-2 inhibitors versus oGLD.

Dapagliflozin Effect on Cardiovascular Events-Thrombolysis in Myocardial Infarction 58 Trial with Dapagliflozin

This trial set out to assess the CV safety of dapagliflozin in patients with T2DM and either established CVD or multiple risk factors. For a median of 4.2 years about 17,160 patients, including >10,000 patients without ASCVD were followed. The mean patient age was 64 years with median diabetes duration of 10.5 years, HbA1c of 8.3%, glomerular filtration rate (GFR) ≥60 mL/min/1.73 m^2, and 40.7% of the patients had established ASCVD. Dapagliflozin met the prespecified criterion for noninferiority to placebo with respect to MACE (upper boundary of the 95% CI, <1.3; p <0.001 for noninferiority) in the primary safety outcome analysis. In the two primary efficacy analyses, dapagliflozin did not result in a lower rate of MACE (8.8% in the dapagliflozin group and 9.4% in the placebo group; HR, 0.93; 95% CI, 0.84–1.03; p = 0.17) but resulted in a lower rate of CV death or HHF (4.9% vs. 5.8%; HR, 0.83; 95% CI, 0.73–0.95; p = 0.005), which reflected a lower rate of HHF (HR, 0.73; 95% CI, 0.61–0.88); there was no between-group difference in CV death (HR, 0.98; 95% CI, 0.82–1.17). The results of this trial indicate that dapagliflozin is superior to placebo in improving glycemic control and noninferior but not superior for reducing MACE in patients with T2DM and high CV risk. There was a reduction in HF hospitalizations, and also a salutary effect on renal outcomes. Unlike canagliflozin, there was no safety signal regarding increased amputations. These are important findings, and more or less consistent with findings noted with other selective inhibitor of SGLT-2 inhibitors.

CLINICAL IMPLICATIONS OF THESE RECENT CARDIOVASCULAR OUTCOME TRIALS WITH SGLT-2 INHIBITORS (FIG. 2)

A recent 2018 meta-analysis published in the Lancet by Marc Sabatine et al. incorporated data from all three randomized controlled trials (RCTs) and deduced that use of SGLT-2 inhibitors caused a statistically significant risk reduction in the 3P-MACE, i.e., MI, stroke, or CV death only in T2DM patients who had pre-existing CVD but not in those who had only multiple risk factors. However, a consistent reduction in risk of HHF as well as renal disease progression was seen in all three trials regardless of the presence of ASCVD or heart failure at baseline. Thus, it can be stated that SGLT-2 inhibitors safely improve glycemic control while reducing the risk of HHF and progression of renal disease across a broad spectrum of patients with T2DM immaterial of presence of established ASCVD or history of heart failure, while incurring the added advantage of reduction in 3P-MACE in patients with established ASCVD. However, there are quite a few differences between the three trial results that cannot be explained as a class effect, bringing forth inconsistencies that await a clear-cut explanation. While canagliflozin and empagliflozin showed a statistically significant 3P-MACE reduction in established

27

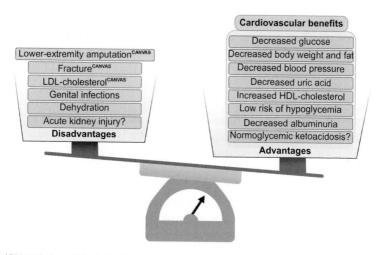

(CANVAS: Canagliflozin Cardiovascular Assessment Study; CV: cardiovascular; DECLARE-TIMI 58: Dapagliflozin Effect on Cardiovascular Events-Thrombolysis in Myocardial Infarction 58; EMPA-REG OUTCOME: Empagliflozin Cardiovascular Outcome Event Trial in Type 2 Diabetes Mellitus Patients; HDL: high-density lipoprotein; LDL: low-density lipoprotein; SGLT-2: sodium-glucose cotransporter-2)

FIG. 2: Advantages and disadvantages in the use of SGLT-2 inhibitors based on CV Outcome Trials.

ASCVD patients, dapagliflozin fell short of it. In similar subgroups, though the CV benefits achieved were almost alike, still in the empagliflozin group, the benefit in CV death reduction in patients with established ASCVD was much more pronounced than with canagliflozin and dapagliflozin. On the other hand, canagliflozin showed an increase in bone fractures and amputations, both empagliflozin and dapagliflozin did not. In the subgroup analysis, Asian patients were not benefited by canagliflozin but rather by empagliflozin and dapagliflozin. The observed variations in CV death may be explained owing to the multiple differences in patient characteristics enrolled in each trial, but subgroup analyses by one variable may not sufficiently capture other important differences.

Furthermore, in patients with lower baseline estimated glomerular filtration rate (eGFR) who are at increased risk for heart failure hospitalizations, the use of SGLT-2 inhibitors by their natriuretic action could be particularly beneficial in reducing progression of renal disease as well as heart failure hospitalizations, accounting for their significant cardiorenal protection in this subgroup and reducing both CV and all-cause mortality. Taken together, the cardiorenal protection offered by this novel class of drugs seems to be a class effect, but further studies are needed to explain for these in-class differences that may not all be attributable to chance. Most importantly play of chance can never be ruled out with data available currently corresponding to one trial with one drug, thus making it prudent to have further additional trials and head-on comparisons between different drugs in the same class to shed further light on this novel class of agents.

CONCLUSION

The Cardiovascular Outcome Trial (CVOT) data from the three landmark SGLT-2 inhibitor trials have dawned a new era in the management strategies for T2DM. The CV effects as well as nephroprotection seen consistently across the group has established these agents as the most promising oral therapies available that offer multiple cardiorenal benefits besides efficacious and durable glycemic control with the added advantage of blood pressure reduction and weight loss. However, individualization of therapy mandates choosing these drugs for the right patient in this era of evidence-based precision medicine so as to minimize the adverse effects.

SUGGESTED READING

1. Fadini GP, Avogaro A. SGLT2 inhibitors and amputations in the US FDA Adverse Event Reporting System. Lancet Diabetes Endocrinol. 2017;5(9):680-1.
2. Koh KK. Letter by Koh Regarding Article, "Randomized Trials to Evaluate Cardiovascular Safety of Antihyperglycemic Medications: A Worthwhile Effort?" Circulation. 2016;134(23):e650-1.
3. Kosiborod M, Cavender MA, Fu AZ, et al. Lower Risk of Heart Failure and Death in Patients Initiated on Sodium-Glucose Cotransporter-2 Inhibitors Versus Other Glucose-Lowering Drugs: The CVD-REAL Study (Comparative Effectiveness of Cardiovascular Outcomes in New Users of Sodium-Glucose Cotransporter-2 Inhibitors). Circulation. 2017;136(3):249-59.
4. Kosiborod M, Lam CS, Kohsaka S, et al. Cardiovascular Events Associated with SGLT-2 Inhibitors Versus Other Glucose-Lowering Drugs: The CVD-REAL 2 Study. J Am Coll Cardiol. 2018;71(23):2628-39.

5. Neal B, Perkovic V, Mahaffey KW, et al. Canagliflozin and Cardiovascular and Renal Events in Type 2 Diabetes. N Engl J Med. 2017;377(7):644-57.
6. Wiviott SD, Raz I, Bonaca MP, et al. Dapagliflozin and Cardiovascular Outcomes in Type 2 Diabetes. N Engl J Med. 2018 [Epub ahead of print].
7. Zelniker TA, Wiviott SD, Raz I, et al. SGLT2 inhibitors for primary and secondary prevention of cardiovascular and renal outcomes in type 2 diabetes: a systematic review and meta-analysis of cardiovascular outcome trials. Lancet. 2018 [Epub ahead of print].
8. Zinman B, Wanner C, Lachin JM, et al. Empagliflozin, Cardiovascular Outcomes, and Mortality in Type 2 Diabetes. N Engl J Med. 2015;373(22):2117-28.

Metabolic and Hemodynamic Effects of SGLT-2 Inhibitors

INTRODUCTION

The inhibition of glucose reabsorption in proximal renal tubules as a result of sodium-glucose cotransporter-2 (SGLT-2) inhibitor action facilitates urinary glucose excretion, translating into a reduction in both fasting and postprandial glucose levels. Improved glucotoxicity with these agents results in an improvement in both pancreatic β-cell function as well as peripheral insulin action. There is a change in whole body energy dynamics to a state of relative glucose deficiency that stimulates lipolysis in adipose tissue as well as fatty acid oxidation and formation of ketone bodies in the liver. Furthermore, these agents have profound hemodynamic effects owing to the increased diuresis, leading to dehydration, reduction in BP as well as weight loss.

Recent clinical trials as well as real-world studies on these new classes of drugs have demonstrated multiple clinical benefits as well as important cardiorenal benefits that have resulted in these agents occupying a much higher place in the hierarchy of antidiabetic therapies. Many hemodynamic and metabolic characteristics of these agents have been proposed on the basis of all these new evidences that have recently emerged pertaining to this unique class of new drugs.

GLYCEMIC EFFICACY OF SODIUM-GLUCOSE COTRANSPORTER-2 INHIBITORS

Treatment with SGLT-2 inhibitors across the class of these agents has shown a consistent improvement in glycemic control, translating into a significant reduction in hemoglobin A1c (HbA1c) as well as fasting and postprandial glucose levels. Larger reductions in HbA1c were seen in patients with poor glycemic control than those with better control. Placebo-adjusted reduction in HbA1c of up to 1.2% has been demonstrated in various studies ranging from 4 weeks to up to 90 weeks duration, both as monotherapy as well as add-on agents to other antidiabetic therapies.

A 2014 meta-analysis showed a greater reduction in HbA1c over 24 weeks with these agents in patients with a lower mean age, shorter diabetes duration, and higher baseline HbA1c, body mass index (BMI) and fasting glucose levels. A randomized, double-blind study of 1,450 patients showed an HbA1c reduction of 0.65% with canagliflozin 100 mg, 0.74% reduction with canagliflozin 300 mg as compared to a 0.55% reduction with glimepiride 6–8 mg over a period of 104 weeks. Further, added benefits to glucose control have been shown when these agents are added to other glucose-lowering therapies—both oral as well as injectable. Dapagliflozin added to patients already on metformin and sulfonylurea showed a decrease in HbA1c of –0.86% compared to a reduction of –0.17% in the placebo group at 24 weeks. Rosenstock et al. demonstrated a marked HbA1c reduction (–0.5 ± 0.1% with 10 mg and –0.6 ± 0.1% with 25 mg, both $p < 0.001$) with empagliflozin in type 2 diabetes patients inadequately controlled on basal insulin in a 78-week randomized, double-blind and placebo-controlled trial. Furthermore, while there was an increment in the basal insulin dose by 5.5 ± 1.6 units in the placebo group, empagliflozin lowered insulin dose requirement by 1.2 ± 1.5 units in the 10 mg group and by 0.5 ± 1.6 units in the 25 mg group, demonstrating that these agents may also reduce insulin dose requirements and mitigate insulin-induced weight gain besides improving glycemic control.

IMPROVEMENTS IN INSULIN SECRETION, INSULIN SENSITIVITY AND GLUCOSE TOXICITY WITH ENHANCED GLUCAGON SECRETION

The metabolic effects of SGLT-2 inhibitors have been a subject of many studies in recent times. Ferrannini et al. measured whole-body glucose utilization using double-tracer glucose administration method after single-dose and chronic empagliflozin 25 mg once daily dosing for 4 weeks compared with baseline levels in 66 patients with type 2 diabetes. Treatment with empagliflozin resulted in urinary glucose excretion—single dose group 7.8 g/3 h and chronic dosing group 9.2 g/3 h during fasting state, and 29 g/5 h and 28.2 g/5 h after a meal, respectively in single dose versus chronic dosing groups. Empagliflozin increased endogenous glucose production by 25% after a 3-hour fast while plasma glucose was significantly lower than baseline. After a meal, endogenous glucose production remained higher in the empagliflozin group compared with the placebo group. In contrast, reductions in both glucose oxidation and nonoxidative glucose disposal lead to significant reduction in the total glucose disposal rate with concomitant increase in lipid oxidation during treatment with empagliflozin. At these metabolic conditions, both glucose and insulin AUCs decreased, whereas the glucagon response increased with empagliflozin treatment after a meal. This strengthens the fact that empagliflozin improves both B-cell function and insulin sensitivity despite a fall in insulin secretion.

In a study by Merovci et al., a similar improvement in muscle insulin sensitivity despite increased fasting glucagon concentration and endogenous glucose production was reported. The study included 18 men with type 2 diabetes, randomized to receive either dapagliflozin (n = 12) or placebo (n = 6) for a duration of 2 weeks. A significant reduction in fasting plasma glucose was noted with dapagliflozin and it also increased insulin-mediated tissue glucose disposal by almost 18% using the hyperinsulinemic glucose clamp technique as shown in previous rodent models. These results provide the first definitive evidence of applicability of glucose toxicity hypothesis to humans with type 2 diabetes.

This interesting phenomenon of paradoxical increases in endogenous glucose production and glucagon secretion despite an overall reduction of fasting plasma glucose after treatment with SGLT-2 inhibition has been comprehensively reviewed. Recent evidence suggests that SGLT-2 is also expressed in glucagon-secreting α-cells of the pancreatic islets, and suppresses glucagon secretion. Chronic hyperglycemia causes downregulation of *SLC5A2* expression, which encodes SGLT-2, with consequent upregulation of glucagon gene expression. Hence treatment with SGLT-2 inhibitors, by suppressing SGLT-2 function in α-cells, might directly cause an increased glucagon secretion from pancreatic α-cells in type 2 diabetes patients with poor glycemic control.

CLINICAL SIGNIFICANCE OF INCREASED KETONE BODY PRODUCTION

An important characteristic of treatment with SGLT-2 inhibitors is an increase in ketone body production. Ketone body production in the liver depends on a relative interaction of action potentials between insulin and its counterregulatory hormones. A relative insufficiency in insulin action versus its counterregulatory hormones increases ketone body production as does a relatively increased action of counterregulatory hormones against insulin. Furthermore, an insufficient glucose intake with a low carbohydrate diet and severe energy restriction, as well as increased glucose energy loss in urine also causes an increase in ketone bodies production. Enhanced glycosuria in patients treated with SGLT-2 inhibitors could result in a relative glucose energy deficit in vivo with a concomitant effective reduction in plasma glucose levels, a concurrent lack of insulin, and an excess of glucagon in plasma, all predisposing to increased ketone body levels.

Recently, the US Food and Drug Administration warned that use of SGLT-2 inhibitors for the treatment of diabetes might lead to an increased risk for diabetic ketoacidosis (DKA) even with mild-to-moderate glucose elevations (euglycemic DKA). Most cases of DKA have been reported in insulin-treated type 2 diabetes patients, more so in those with insulinopenia or in a severe catabolic state such as sepsis or suffering from an intercurrent illness. A recent review article reported the incidence of DKA to be <0.1% in the clinical trials using dapagliflozin [Dapagliflozin Effect on Cardiovascular Events (DECLARE)], empagliflozin [Empagliflozin Cardiovascular Outcome Event Trial in Type 2 Diabetes Mellitus Patients (EMPA-REG OUTCOME)], and canagliflozin [Canagliflozin Cardiovascular Assessment Study (CANVAS)], and in the other published reports in both patients with type 1 and type 2 diabetes. Thus, it is pertinent that all patients with insulin-treated diabetes who develop nausea, vomiting and malaise during treatment with

SGLT-2 inhibitors should be promptly evaluated for the possible occurrence of ketoacidosis even in conditions of euglycemia or mild hyperglycemia.

HEMODYNAMIC AND RENAL EFFECTS WITH BLOOD PRESSURE LOWERING ACTION OF SGLT-2 INHIBITORS

The prevalence of cardiovascular diseases (CVDs) is much higher in people with type 2 diabetes than nondiabetics. Both hypertension and diabetes are major risk factors for CVD, and both are frequently seen to coexist. Furthermore, up to 75% of CVD in diabetes is attributable to hypertension, thus making a case for aggressive hypertension management in such patients in addition to glucose-lowering. Besides, blood pressure lowering also has renoprotective effects in patients with T2DM. The use of SGLT-2 inhibitors has demonstrated a significant reduction in blood pressure—2.8 mm Hg systolic and 1.6 mm Hg diastolic, respectively in a pooled analysis of five randomized controlled trials. The potential mechanisms for blood pressure-lowering action of these agents include osmotic diuresis, natriuresis as well as increased degradation of adipose tissue and muscle mass and body weight reduction, though further studies are awaited to fully elucidate the exact mechanisms leading to blood pressure reductions and increased hematocrit with SGLT-2 inhibitors.

CARDIOVASCULAR BENEFITS: IMPLICATIONS OF THE CARDIOVASCULAR OUTCOME TRIALS

Although cardiovascular mortality is established as a principal cause of death in patients with T2DM, glucose lowering does not have a major effect on reducing CVD risk. SGLT-2 inhibitors are a novel class of antihyperglycemic agents that have shown cardiorenal benefits in addition to glucose control and blood pressure reduction and weight loss. The three landmark cardiovascular outcome trials with empagliflozin, canagliflozin and dapagliflozin have established these agents as oral drugs of choice in patients with atherosclerotic cardiovascular disease (ASCVD).

In the EMPA-REG OUTCOME Trial, 7,020 patients with long-standing type 2 diabetes (>10 years in 57% of the patients) with a mean age of 63 years at high risk of CVDs with >99% patients having established CVD (76% had coronary artery disease, 47% had history of myocardial infarction), were randomly assigned into three groups (placebo, empagliflozin 10 mg/day, and empagliflozin 25 mg/day), and were followed for a median of 3.1 years. Mean baseline HbA1c was 8.1%. Background diabetes treatment was first unchanged for 12 weeks. Placebo-adjusted mean reductions in HbA1c in the empagliflozin treatment groups were –0.54% at 12 weeks and –0.24% at 206 weeks. The primary endpoints defined as three-point major adverse cardiovascular events (3P-MACE) included death from cardiovascular causes, nonfatal myocardial infarction, and nonfatal stroke. The trial showed a primary composite of 3P-MACE reduction by 14% (p <0.001 for noninferiority; p = 0.04 for superiority). With no significant reduction in the relative risk of stroke or myocardial infarction this MACE risk reduction was primarily driven by a 38% relative risk reduction in cardiovascular death [hazard ratio (HR), 0.62; 95% confidence interval (CI), 0.49–0.77; p <0.001]. Furthermore, there was a 32% relative risk reduction in all-cause mortality (HR, 0.68; 95% CI, 0.57–0.82; p <0.001) and a 35% relative risk reduction in the incidence of hospitalization for heart failure (HR, 0.65; 95% CI, 0.50–0.85; p = 0.002).

The CANVAS Program integrated data from two trials involving a total of 10,142 participants with type 2 diabetes and either established CVD or those at high cardiovascular risk. The mean age of the participants was 63.3 years, 35.8% were women, the mean duration of diabetes was 13.5 years, and 65.6% had an established history of CVD. Participants in each trial were randomly assigned to receive canagliflozin 100 mg or 300 mg daily or placebo and were followed for a mean of 188.2 weeks. The primary outcome was a composite of death from cardiovascular causes, nonfatal myocardial infarction, or nonfatal stroke. The rate of the primary outcome was lower with canagliflozin than with placebo (occurring in 26.9 participants vs 31.5 participants per 1,000 patient-years; HR, 0.86; 95% CI, 0.75–0.97; p <0.001 for noninferiority; p = 0.02 for superiority). Nearly 34% of the cohort was enrolled for primary prevention (age ≥50 years, no known coronary artery disease/

CVD/ peripheral artery disease, at least two risk factors). The secondary prevention subset had higher event rates. Canagliflozin, as compared with placebo, reduced the primary endpoint (p = 0.18), heart failure hospitalization (p = 0.91), and progression to albuminuria (p = 0.48) in both subgroups. It also increased lower extremity amputations (p = 0.63) in both subgroups.

The Dapagliflozin Effect on Cardiovascular Events-Thrombolysis in Myocardial Infarction 58 (DECLARE-TIMI 58) set out to assess the cardiovascular safety of dapagliflozin in patients with T2DM and either established CVD or multiple risk factors. A total of 17,160 patients, including 10,186 patients without ASCVD were followed for a median of 4.2 years. The mean patient age was 64 years with median diabetes duration of 10.5 years, HbA1c of 8.3%, glomerular filtration rate (GFR) $\geq$60 mL/min/1.73 m^2, and 40.7% of the patients had established ASCVD. In the primary safety outcome analysis, dapagliflozin met the prespecified criterion for noninferiority to placebo with respect to MACE (upper boundary of the 95% CI, <1.3; p <0.001 for noninferiority). In the two primary efficacy analyses, dapagliflozin did not result in a lower rate of MACE (8.8% in the dapagliflozin group and 9.4% in the placebo group; HR, 0.93; 95% CI, 0.84–1.03; p = 0.17) but did result in a lower rate of cardiovascular death or hospitalization for heart failure (4.9% vs 5.8%; HR, 0.83; 95% CI, 0.73–0.95; p = 0.005), which reflected a lower rate of hospitalization for heart failure (HR, 0.73; 95% CI, 0.61–0.88); there was no between-group difference in cardiovascular death (HR, 0.98; 95% CI, 0.82–1.17). The results of this trial indicate that dapagliflozin is superior to placebo in improving glycemic control and noninferior but not superior for reducing MACE in patients with T2DM and high cardiovascular risk. There was a reduction in heart failure hospitalizations, and also a salutary effect on renal outcomes. Unlike canagliflozin, there was no safety signal regarding increased amputations. These are important findings, and more or less consistent with findings noted with other selective inhibitor of SGLT-2 inhibitors.

A recent meta-analysis published in the Lancet by Marc Sabatine et al. incorporated data from all three randomized controlled trials (RCTs) and showed that use of SGLT-2 inhibitors were clinically beneficial in reducing the risk of myocardial infarction, stroke or cardiovascular death only in T2DM patients with established CVD and not in those with multiple risk factors. However, a significant reduction in risk of hospitalizations for heart failure as well as renal disease progression was seen regardless of the presence of ASCVD or heart failure at baseline. This offers us important clinical insights into the fact that SGLT-2 inhibitors safely improve glycemic control while reducing the risk of hospitalization for heart failure and progression of renal disease across a broad spectrum of patients with T2DM regardless of presence of ASCVD or history of heart failure, with the added advantage of reduction in MACE in patients with established ASCVD.

The unprecedented CV benefits that these agents incur have led to a number of hypotheses being proposed as possible mechanisms behind these effects of which the two most likely mechanisms are as follows:

1. Hemodynamic effects including blood pressure lowering, diuresis and increased hematocrit
2. Metabolic effects relating to negative glucose and energy balance including ketone body production, and reduction in atherogenic risk factors including decrease in HbA1c, body weight, uric acid and triglyceride, as well as increase in high-density lipoprotein cholesterol (HDL-C) (Fig. 1).

Ferranini et al. and Mudaliar et al. looked into the metabolic dynamics of substrate utilization in diabetes and/or heart failure to explain the early and consistent cardiorenal benefits seen from as early as 3 months of commencing SGLT-2 inhibitor therapy. It has been established that in diabetes as well as in heart failure, the metabolic flexibility of the heart in terms of substrate utilization is impaired. They postulated that the mild persistent hyperketonemia induced by SGLT-2 inhibitors induces the myocardium as well as other organs including the kidneys to freely take up this beta-hydroxybutyrate (βOHB) as a preferential substrate—"superfuel"—over nonesterified fatty acids (NEFAs) and glucose. This fuel selection improves the transduction of oxygen consumption into work efficiency at the level of mitochondria. Experiments have shown that in the isolated working heart, βOHB simultaneously increases external cardiac work while reducing oxygen consumption, thereby improving cardiac efficiency by 24%. Thus, the failing heart turns to using ketones rather than fatty

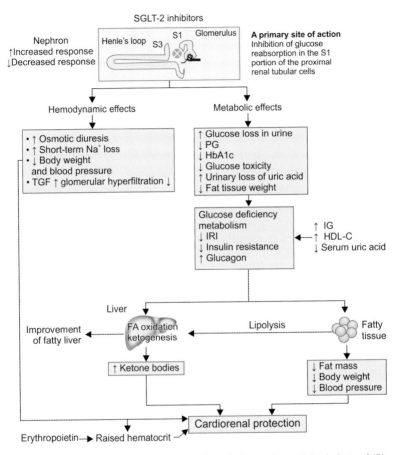

(FA: fatty acid; HbA1c: hemoglobin A1c; HDL-C: high-density lipoprotein cholesterol; IRI: immunoreactive insulin)

FIG. 1: Multifactorial metabolic and hemodynamic effects of sodium-glucose cotransporter-2 (SGLT-2) inhibitors to protect cardiorenal outcomes. S1 portion of the proximal renal tubular cells is specifically the primary site of action for SGLT-2 inhibitors, they inhibit Na+/glucose cotransport and hence the increased urinary glucose loss. The main parts of these multifactorial effects are shown: (i) reduction of plasma glucose, insulin, body fat mass, as well as body weight, (ii) osmotic diuresis and loop diuretic action with reductions of body weight and blood pressure, and activation of tubuloglomerular feedback (TGF) mechanisms with consequently decreased glomerular hyperfiltration. In addition to those effects, increased plasma glucagon secretion is directly activated with the SGLT-2 inhibitor treatment. Increased hematocrit is possibly related to erythropoietin secretion with an unknown mechanism and serum uric acid is also reduced.

acids to cope with the increased energy expenditure. Furthermore, in vitro systems have also demonstrated suppression of oxidative stress by βOHB-induced inhibition of histone deacetylases. Finally, ketone bodies have also been shown to upregulate mitochondrial biogenesis and exhibit antiarrhythmic potential by stabilizing cell membrane potential. Moreover, the hemoconcentration manifested by a raised hematocrit (secondary to diuresis or may be stimulation of erythropoiesis) by SGLT-2 inhibition increases oxygen delivery to the tissues, establishing a powerful synergy with the substrate shift in a metabolically flexible heart.

The concept that SGLT-2 inhibitors reduced cardiovascular events primarily through prevention of heart failure (vs. atherothrombotic events) has gained broad acceptance after rapidly accumulating evidences. Studies in nondiabetics have also exhibited glucosuria, natriuresis, increased glucagon levels as well as ketone bodies with these agents. It is not wrong in hypothesizing that similar cardiorenal benefits may be observed in nondiabetics as well and this is a hot topic of exploration in various ongoing heart failure studies with dapagliflozin as well as empagliflozin in this group. As our understanding of these agents improves, mechanistic hypotheses accounting for their remarkable cardioprotective action include potential effects on myocardial metabolism, direct effects on myocardium and adipokine kinetics besides effects on volume, and diuresis for further exploration. A state of the art review published recently in Diabetologia elucidates the various proposed mechanisms for cardiovascular benefits with SGLT-2 inhibitors as here:

- Improvement in ventricular loading conditions by causing a reduction in preload (secondary to natriuresis and osmotic diuresis) and afterload (reduction in blood pressure along with an improvement in vascular function). Certain unique features separate these agents from traditional diuretics including their ability to selectively reduce interstitial fluid and this may limit the reflex neurohumoral stimulation that occurs in response to intravascular volume contraction with traditional diuretics as well as their uricosuric action in contrast to conventional diuretics that increase uric acid levels, possible affecting cardiovascular outcomes. Studies have also demonstrated an improvement in endothelial function and aortic stiffness indices with use of SGLT-2 inhibitors as well as potential induction of vasodilatation by activation of voltage-gated potassium (Kv) channels and protein kinase G

- *Improvement in cardiac metabolism and bioenergetics*: As explained earlier, SGLT-2 inhibitors are known to slightly increase the production of the ketone body βOHB. Ferranini et al. hypothesized that this may be the "superfuel" offering an alternative and less expensive fuel source to the myocardium in place of NEFAs or glucose, not only improving cardiac function in the failing heart, but also increasing mechanical efficiency. Others have postulated that SGLT-2 inhibitor-induced increase in βOHB levels may prevent prohypertrophic transcription pathways by inhibiting histone deacetylase. Also, a reduction in βOHB oxidation results in decreased acetyl-CoA derived from ketone oxidation, thereby increasing the oxidation of glucose-derived pyruvate implying an improvement in myocardial glucose metabolism. Also, the reduction in acetyl-CoA supply may also decrease harmful hyperacetylation of mitochondrial enzymes, thereby improving mitochondrial energy production

- *Myocardial Na^+/H^+ exchange inhibition*: Experimental heart failure models have shown an increase in cytosolic sodium and calcium levels secondary to activation of the Na^+/H^+ exchanger (NHE) 1 isoform in the myocardium. It has been demonstrated that empagliflozin causes inhibition of cardiomyocyte NHE reducing cytoplasmic sodium and calcium levels while increasing calcium levels in the mitochondria. This has lead to an emerging hypothesis of direct inhibitory action of SGLT-2 inhibitors on the myocardial NHE1 isoform

- *Reduction of necrosis and cardiac fibrosis*: Cardiac fibrosis involving cardiac structural remodeling by deposition of extracellular matrix proteins by cardiac fibroblasts results in impairment of ventricular compliance and accelerates development of heart failure. Various preliminary experimental studies in rat models as well as human cardiac fibroblasts have shown antifibrotic effects of dapagliflozin as well as empagliflozin through direct and favorable effects on cardiac fibroblast phenotype and function, contributing to their possibly favorable effects in reducing heart failure

41

- *Alteration in adipokines, cytokine production and epicardial adipose tissue mass*: Altered paracrine regulation of adipokines on the myocardium resulting in ectopic fat deposition (perivascular and epicardial) has been implicated in the pathogenesis of heart failure. There is now emerging suggestion that SGLT-2 inhibitors may have a role in reducing proinflammatory adipokines such as leptin that may have a role in cardiac inflammation and fibrosis, as well as decreasing inflammatory cytokine interleukin-6 (IL-6) as well as increasing levels of anti-inflammatory adipokines like adiponectin.

RENAL BENEFITS

The abovementioned three landmark RCTs on SGLT-2 inhibitors besides showing cardiovascular benefits also demonstrated renoprotective effects in patients with T2DM. The Sabatine et al. in Lancet 2018 meta-analysis endorsed this renoprotection, showing an overall 45% reduction in the composite of renal function worsening, end-stage renal disease or renal death (HR, 0.55; 95% CI, 0.48–0.64; p <0.0001). Interestingly, the renal benefits were robust both in the patients with established ASCVD (HR, 0.56; 95% CI, 0.47–0.67) and those with multiple risk factors (HR, 0.54; 95% CI, 0.42–0.71), p for interaction = 0.71. Furthermore, this reduction in renal composite was seen across the spectrum of estimated glomerular filtration rate (eGFR) levels but was highest in those with preserved renal function at baseline, with a 33% reduction in patients with an eGFR <60 mL/min/1.73 m^2, 44% reduction in those with an eGFR 60–90 mL/min/1.73 m^2, and a 56% reduction in those with an eGFR ≥90 mL/min/1.73 m^2. Patients with worse baseline renal function showed a much better reduction in heart failure hospitalizations with these drugs than the reduction in renal composite which may be explained with the natriuresis induced by these drugs in addition to their renoprotective effects as this subgroup are actually at an increased risk for heart failure hospitalization. These reductions in both kidney disease progression as well as hospitalization for heart failure and their attendant interventions and proceeding complications may eventually reduce the risk for CV death and all-cause death seen with SGLT-2 inhibitors (Fig. 2).

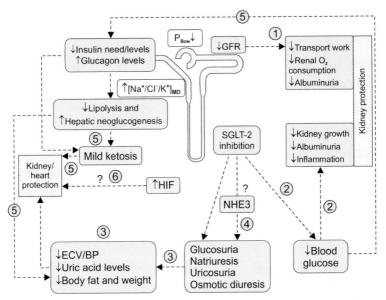

(ECV: extracellular volume; GFR: glomerular filtration rate; HIF: hypoxia-inducible factor; NHE3: sodium-hydrogen antiporter 3; SGLT-2: sodium-glucose cotransporter-2)

FIG. 2: A summary of possible mechanisms of renal protection associated with SGLT-2 inhibitors. The pleiotropic effects of SGLT-2 inhibition may provide cardioprotective and renal protective effects via several mechanisms: (1) SGLT-2 inhibition attenuates primary proximal tubular hyperreabsorption in the kidney in diabetes, increasing/restoring the tubuloglomerular feedback signal at the macula densa [$(Na^+/Cl^-/K^+)_{MD}$] and hydrostatic pressure in Bowman's space (P_{Bow}). This reduces glomerular hyperfiltration, beneficially affecting albumin filtration and tubular transport work, and thus, renal oxygen consumption; (2) By lowering blood glucose levels, SGLT-2 inhibitors can reduce kidney growth, albuminuria, and inflammation; (3) SGLT-2 inhibitors have a modest osmotic, diuretic, natriuretic and uricosuric effect, which can reduce ECV, blood pressure, serum uric acid levels and body weight. These changes may have beneficial effects on both the renal and cardiovascular systems; (4) SGLT-2 may be functionally linked to NHE3, such that SGLT-2 inhibition may also inhibit NHE3 in the proximal tubule, with implications on the natriuretic, GFR, and blood pressure effect; (5) SGLT-2 inhibition reduces insulin levels and the need for therapeutic or endogenous insulin and increases glucagon levels. As a consequence, lipolysis and hepatic gluconeogenesis are elevated. These metabolic adaptations reduce fat tissue/ body weight and hypoglycemia risk, and result in mild ketosis, potentially having beneficial effects on both the renal and cardiovascular systems; (6) SGLT-2 inhibition may also enhance renal HIF content, which may have renal protective effects. Pink text boxes indicate affected variables; white text boxes indicate processes that link SGLT-2 inhibition to the reduction in GFR. Dash arrows demonstrate consequences; solid arrows indicate changes in associated variables (increase/decrease).

There have been multifactorial potential mechanisms that may explain these renal benefits, with direct renovascular as well as hemodynamic effects postulated to have a key role in nephroprotection by SGLT-2 inhibition (Fig. 3). The reduction

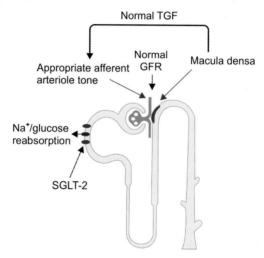

A   **Normal physiology**

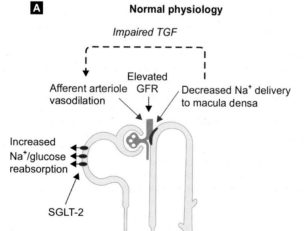

B   **Hyperfiltration in early stages
of diabetic nephropathy**

Continued

Continued

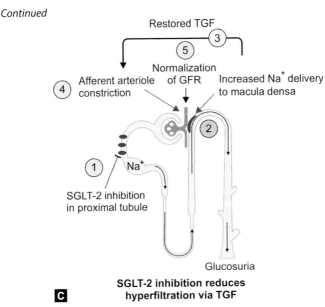

SGLT-2 inhibition reduces hyperfiltration via TGF

(GFR: glomerular filtration rate; SGLT-2: sodium-glucose cotransporter-2; TGF: tubulo-glomerular feedback)

FIG. 3: Possible renal hemodynamic effects associated with SGLT-2 inhibition. (A) Under physiological conditions, TGF signaling maintains stable GFR by modulation of preglomerular arteriole tone. In case of conditional increase in GFR, the macula densa within the juxtaglomerular apparatus senses an increase in distal tubular sodium delivery and adjusts GFR via TGF accordingly; (B) Under chronic hyperglycemic conditions (diabetes mellitus), increased proximal SGLT-2-mediated reabsorption of sodium (Na^+) glucose impairs this feedback mechanism. Thus, despite increased GFR, the macula densa is exposed to lowered sodium concentrations. This impairment of TGF signaling likely leads to inadequate arteriole tone and increased renal perfusion; (C) SGLT-2 inhibition with empagliflozin treatment blocks proximal tubule glucose and sodium reabsorption, which leads to increased sodium delivery to the macula densa. This condition restores TGF via appropriate modulation of arteriolar tone (e.g. afferent vasoconstriction), which, in turn, reduces renal plasma flow and hyperfiltration.

in proximal tubular sodium reabsorption caused by these drugs causes an increased delivery of sodium to the macula densa, thus activating the tubuloglomerular feedback leading to afferent arteriolar vasoconstriction and reduced renal blood flow, finally reducing the glomerular hyperfiltration. Also, SGLT-2 inhibition has been shown to improve intraglomerular hypertension in patients with T1DM and hyperfiltration. These renal hemodynamic changes that result in reduction in glomerular hyperfiltration and reduction in intraglomerular pressure clinically manifest as acute reduction in eGFR and albuminuria which is eventually followed up epidermal growth factor receptor (EGFR) stabilization translating into long-term renal benefits. The multifactorial proposed mechanisms contributing to nephroprotection by these drugs include the modest diuresis along with BP reduction, reduction in HbA1c and body weight as well as their uricosuric action. Furthermore, protection from renal tubular hypoxia through increased ketogenesis and an increased hematocrit have also been elucidated as possible contributors to long-term renal benefits observed with these agents.

CONCLUSION

The advent of SGLT-2 inhibitors into the arena of antidiabetic therapies has changed the paradigms of diabetes management. Besides their insulin-independent glucose-lowering efficacy, glucosuria induced by these agents induces a negative glucose energy balance and they also increase fatty acid oxidation and increase ketone body production. They improve glucotoxicity by improving insulin secretion and insulin sensitivity. The diuresis and natriuresis resulting by their use induces both BP reduction and weight loss, and leads to an increased hematocrit by yet to be explained mechanisms. The dramatic renal benefits in addition to the cardiovascular benefits demonstrated by these agents in the landmark EMPA-REG OUTCOME trial, CANVAS program and the DECLARE-TIMI 58 trial have placed these agents much higher in the diabetes management algorithms as our understanding of their unique metabolic and hemodynamic mechanisms still keeps improving in this era of evidence-based medicine.

SUGGESTED READING

1. Cefalu WT, Stenlöf K, Leiter LA, et al. Effects of canagliflozin on body weight and relationship to HbA1c and blood pressure changes in patients with type 2 diabetes. Diabetologia. 2015;58(6):1183-7.

2. Cefalu WT. Paradoxical insights into whole body metabolic adaptations following SGLT2 inhibition. J Clin Invest. 2014;124(2):485-7.
3. Chao EC. SGLT2 Inhibitors: A New Mechanism for Glycemic Control. Clin Diabetes. 2014;32(1):4-11.
4. Ferrannini E, Baldi S, Frascerra S, et al. Shift to Fatty Substrate Utilization in Response to Sodium-Glucose Cotransporter 2 Inhibition in Subjects Without Diabetes and Patients With Type 2 Diabetes. Diabetes. 2016;65(5):1190-5.
5. Ferrannini E, Mark M, Mayoux E. CV protection in the EMPA-REG OUTCOME Trial: A "Thrifty Substrate" Hypothesis. Diabetes Care. 2016;39(7):1108-14.
6. Merovci A, Solis Herrera C, Daniele G, et al. Dapagliflozin improves muscle insulin sensitivity but enhances endogenous glucose production. J Clin Invest. 2014;124:509-14.
7. Monami M, Nardini C, Mannucci E. Efficacy and safety of sodium glucose co-transport-2 inhibitors in type 2 diabetes: a meta-analysis of randomized clinical trials. Diabetes Obes Metab. 2014;16(5):457-66.
8. Mudaliar S, Alloju S, Henry RR. Can a Shift in Fuel Energetics Explain the Beneficial Cardiorenal Outcomes in the EMPA-REG OUTCOME Study? A Unifying Hypothesis. Diabetes Care. 2016;39(7):1115-22.
9. Neal B, Perkovic V, Mahaffey KW, et al. Canagliflozin and Cardiovascular and Renal Events in Type 2 Diabetes. N Engl J Med. 2017;377(7):644-57.
10. Peters AL, Buschur EO, Buse JB, et al. Euglycemic Diabetic Ketoacidosis: A Potential Complication of Treatment With Sodium-Glucose Cotransporter 2 Inhibition. Diabetes Care. 2015;38(9):1687-93.
11. Rosenstock J, Ferrannini E. Euglycemic Diabetic Ketoacidosis: A Predictable, Detectable, and Preventable Safety Concern with SGLT2 Inhibitors. Diabetes Care. 2015;38(9):1638-42.
12. Verma S, McMurray JJ. SGLT2 inhibitors and mechanisms of cardiovascular benefit: a state-of-the-art review. Diabetologia. 2018;61(10):2108-17.
13. Wanner C. EMPA-REG OUTCOME: The Nephrologist's Point of View. Am J Med. 2017;130(6S):S63-72.
14. Wiviott SD, Raz I, Bonaca MP, et al. Dapagliflozin and Cardiovascular Outcomes in Type 2 Diabetes. N Engl J Med. 2018. [Epub ahead of print].
15. Zelniker TA, Wiviott SD, Raz I, et al. SGLT2 inhibitors for primary and secondary prevention of cardiovascular and renal outcomes in type 2 diabetes: a systematic review and meta-analysis of cardiovascular outcome trials. Lancet. 2018. [Epub ahead of print].
16. Zinman B, Wanner C, Lachin JM, et al. Empagliflozin, Cardiovascular Outcomes, and Mortality in Type 2 Diabetes. N Engl J Med. 2015;373(22):2117-28.

Adverse Effects and Safety of SGLT-2 Inhibitors

INTRODUCTION

Sodium-glucose cotransporter-2 (SGLT-2) inhibitors are fast emerging as very efficacious agents for management of type 2 diabetes mellitus (T2DM) more so with their pleiotropic benefits of weight loss, blood pressure (BP) reduction as well as cardiovascular (CV) and renal benefits. As a result their acceptability as antidiabetic drugs is fast improving and most guidelines today place them much higher in the hierarchy as choice of preferred agents for diabetes control. Though these drugs have multiple benefits, they do come with their own share of side effects and safety issues one has to be vigilant about. The most frequently reported adverse events such as euglycemic diabetic ketoacidosis (DKA), urinary tract infections (UTIs), genital mycotic infections, etc. have been reported as a class effect with these agents, while others such as lower limb amputations, bone effects, etc. have been observed in specifically with canagliflozin and not much with the other agents, raising speculation on intra-class differences between different drugs in this group. Concerns have also been raised in terms of declining renal function, acute kidney injury with these drugs. This chapter covers the safety profile and reported adverse events with these agents while looking at the various explanations for these reported side effects. A thorough knowledge of these issues can enable the reader to individualize treatment in choosing the right patient for this very potent class of new drugs to minimize these undesired side effects.

HYPOGLYCEMIA

Almost all glucose-lowering therapies run the risk of causing hypo-glycemia, making it the most limiting factor in achieving target glycemic control. Besides the increased CV risk associated with hypoglycemia, poor compliance and weight gain due to defensive eating because of fear of hypoglycemia worsen the quality of life for diabetic patients. SGLT-2 inhibitors per se do not induce hypoglycemia due to various mechanistic factors. They reduce glucotoxicity and improve insulin resistance resulting in reduced insulin secretion from pancreatic β-cells. The excess glucosuria induced by SGLT-2 inhibitor action is limited by increased SGLT-1-mediated glucose reabsorption at the proximal tubules. Also, by their direct effect on pancreatic α-cells as well as reduced glucose levels, SGLT-2 inhibitors stimulate glucagon secretion, which further prevents hypoglycemia by increasing hepatic glucose production.

However, coadministration of these drugs with potent hypo-glycemic agents such as sulfonylureas has been shown to increase the risk of hypoglycemia though this was not documented with metformin or insulin. This makes it sensible to reduce the dose of sulfonylureas or even insulin by 10–20% when SGLT-2 inhibitors are initiated to prevent hypoglycemia in such patients.

GENITAL TRACT INFECTIONS

The SGLT-2 inhibitors work by inducing glucosuria which helps in normalizing glucose levels. The increased glucose content in urine has the potential to increase fungal growth especially in the genitourinary tract and perineum, predisposing the patients to increased risk for genital mycotic infections. The use of all three gliflozins—empagliflozin, dapagliflozin as well as canagliflozin-has been associated with an increased risk of genital tract infections (GTIs) ranging between 5–15% in different clinical trials. The risk is more in females than males (4–5 times) manifesting most commonly as mycotic vulvovaginitis in women and as mycotic balanitis or balanoposthitis in men. *Candida* species, more commonly *Candida glabrata* is the most commonly associated pathogen in most patients. GTIs are more frequent in individuals with a history of genital infections and are not influenced by HbA1c levels. Generally these can be treated by standard course of antibiotics/antifungals and do not recur, hence in most cases drug discontinuation is not required. It is essential the perineal hygiene be maintained along with adequate hydration when prescribing these drugs to patients and these should be avoided in patients with recurrent upper UTIs, complicated GTIs as well as refractory urinary as well as GTIs.

URINARY TRACT INFECTIONS

The use of SGLT-2 inhibitors is also purported to slightly increase the risk for UTIs, though GTIs are more common. Hyperglycemia per se increases UTI risk owing to multiple factors such as glucosuria, immune dysfunction, increased adherence of bacteria to urothelium as well as increased estrogen levels. SGLT-2 inhibitors, by increasing glucosuria in uncontrolled T2DM further accentuate this risk and may be associated with mild-to-moderate UTI, though generally these care easily treated with standard course of antibiotics and do not recur. Severe complicated and upper UTIs such as pyelonephritis have also been reported, though rare.

Large clinical trials with these drugs have shown variable results (Table 1). In CANVAS, canagliflozin showed increase in GTIs—34.9 events per 1,000 patient years versus 10.8 events per 1,000 patient years in males (p <0.001) as well as 68.8 events per 1,000 patient years versus 17.5 events per 1,000 patient years in females (p <0.001). In contrast, no increase in UTIs was seen with canagliflozin (40 events per 1,000 patient years with canagliflozin versus 37 events per 1,000 patient years in the placebo arm (p = 0.38). Similarly in EMPA-REG the GTIs, mainly in women, were increased in the empagliflozin arm versus the placebo arm (6.4% vs. 1.8% respectively, p <0.05), while the UTIs were similar in both groups (18% in the empagliflozin arm vs. 18.1% in the placebo arm). Even the rates of complicated UTIs were similar in both groups—1.7% in the empagliflozin arm and 1.8% in the placebo arm. Even DECLARE showed similar rates of UTIs in dapagliflozin arm and placebo arm (1.5% and 1.6% respectively) while GTIs were significantly increased in the dapagliflozin arm versus placebo arm (0.9% vs. 0.1% respectively, p <0.001). Thus all three completed randomized controlled trials (RCTs) with SGLT-2 inhibitors showed increased GTIs while no significant increase in

TABLE 1: Effect of sodium-glucose linked transporter type 2 (SGLT-2) inhibitors on urinary tract infections.

STUDY (Type)	Sample size (n)	Agent used	Results
EMPA-REG OUTCOME (RCT)	7,020	Empagliflozin	No increased risk of UTI was seen (18.1%in the placebo group vs.18% in the study group)
CANVAS (RCT)	10,142	Canagliflozin	No increased risk of UTI was seen (40 events per 1,000 patient years in the study group vs. 37 events per 1,000 patient years in the placebo group, p = 0.38)
Kawalec et al. (Meta-analysis)	1,150	Dapagliflozin and Canagliflozin	As compared with placebo, no increased risk of UTI (RR 1.02, 95% CI 0.54–1.91)
Li et al. (Meta-analysis)	36,689	All SGLT-2 inhibitors	No increased risk of UTI except for dapagliflozin (OR 1.28, 95% CI 1.06–1.54)
Liu et al. (Meta-analysis)	50,820	All SGLT-2 inhibitors	No increased risk of UTI was seen (RR for SGLT-2 inhibitors 1.05, 95% CI 0.98–1.12) Only dapagliflozin was associated with increased risk of UTI (RR 1.34, 95% CI 1.11–1.63)
Vasilakou et al. (Meta-analysis)	16,407	All SGLT-2 inhibitors	UTI more commonly seen in patients receiving SGLT-2 inhibitors (OR 1.34, 95% CI 1.03–1.74)
Yang et al. (Meta-analysis)	3,669	All SGLT-2 inhibitors	No increased risk of UTI was seen (OR 1.34, 95% CI 0.79–2.27)
Zaccardi et al. (Meta-analysis)	23,997	All SGLT-2 inhibitors	Only dapagliflozin was associated with increased risk of UTI as compared to placebo (OR 1.32,95% CI 1.06–1.63)

UTIs was seen. On the other hand various individual studies with these agents as well as meta-analyses have reported increased UTIs with these agents. Severe UTIs including acute pyelonephritis have been rarely described, making it important to observe caution in prescribing SGLT-2 inhibitors in male patients with urinary tract outlet obstruction where severe UTIs have been reported with these agents.

EUGLYCEMIC DIABETIC KETOACIDOSIS

A very controversial adverse event seen with SGLT-2 inhibitors that the USFDA in its drug safety communication warned about is an increase in the risk of DKA with this drug on a background of uncharacteristically mild-to-moderate glucose elevations (euglycemic DKA). Though FDA did acknowledge that most cases did occur where the drug was used off-label in T1DM patients, yet its occurrence in T2DM patients has been well documented. T2DM who developed this complication were mostly hospitalized patients in a catabolic state or with severe sepsis, indicating certain red flags we need to be careful about when prescribing this drug.

Traditionally DKA generally occurs in states of absolute insulin deficiency leading to reduced glucose utilization and increased lipolysis that increased free fatty acid influx into the liver which in the background of increased glucagon levels get oxidized to produce ketone bodies. Ketosis also results as a result of severe dietary carbohydrate restriction that prompts an increased dependence on fat oxidation for energy needs, further enhancing ketogenesis. The euglycemic DKA, with plasma glucose levels <300 mg/dL. It has been reported with these agents in T1DM patients (two-thirds of whom were females) has been attributed to a reduced insulin dosage with reduced carbohydrate consumption which prompted lipolysis in these patients. On the other hand, in T2DM patients, it was more attributed to the mechanism of action of drug which by inducing rapid glucosuria (50–100 g/day), reduces plasma glucose levels and consequently insulin secretion and stimulates glucagon production at mild to moderately elevated glucose levels, increasing lipolysis and ketone body production. This was exaggerated in T2DM patients with severe sepsis or in a catabolic state or on carbohydrate restriction, who were on an SGLT-2 inhibitor, increasing ketogenesis in such patients, more-so in those with some degree of insulinopenia, resulting in euglycemic DKA.

A study in drug-naïve or metformin treated well controlled T2DM patients on SGLT-2 inhibitors showed a plasma glucose reduction of 20–25 mg/dL in both overnight fasting as well as post-mixed meal state and a consequent fall in plasma insulin levels (by ~10 pmol/L fasting and ~60 pmol/L postmeal). There was a significant increase in plasma glucagon concentrations owing partly to the diminished paracrine insulin inhibition as well as reduced SGLT-2- mediated glucose transport into α-cells. This caused a drop in the calculated insulin-to-glucagon molar concentration ratio from 9 to 7 mol/mol in the fasting state and from 29 to 24 mol/mol during the meal, releasing the inhibition of hepatic neoglucogenesis and increasing endogenous glucose production both in the fasting as well as postmeal state. The reduction in glucotoxicity also lead to an improvement in insulin sensitivity as demonstrated using the euglycemic insulin clamp.

Few pathophysiological characteristics as depicted in Figure 1 below differentiate the SGLT-2 inhibitor-induced euDKA from

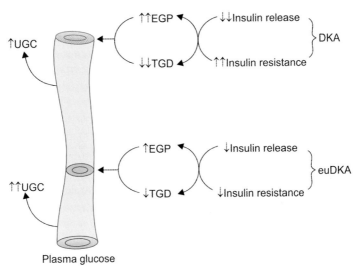

(TGD: tissue glucose disposal; UGC: urinary glucose clearance rate; EGP: endogenous glucose production; DKA: diabetic ketoacidosis; euDKA: euglycemic diabetic ketoacidosis)

FIG. 1: Making DKA. Essential pathophysiology of DKA and euDKA consequent of the use of SGLT-2 inhibitors.

conventional DKA. In euDKA the insulin deficiency as well as insulin resistance are milder and hence the glucose overproduction and underutilization are markedly lesser than in DKA. Furthermore, the renal glucose clearance, i.e. the ratio of glucosuria to prevailing glycemia in euDKA is almost double than that seen in DKA.

BLOOD PRESSURE CHANGES

The BP lowering effect of SGLT-2 inhibitors has been well established and hypothesized to be due to chronic osmotic diuresis, natriuresis, changes in nitric oxide release as well as reduced arterial stiffness, demonstrating dose-related increases in 24-hour urinary volumes between 100 mL and 470 mL. Dapagliflozin studies have demonstrated up to 5 mm Hg systolic blood pressure (SBP) reduction with DECLARE-TIMI showing a 2.7 mm Hg reduction in SBP and 0.7 mm Hg diastolic blood pressure (DBP) reduction. Similarly, canagliflozin caused a 3.93 mm Hg reduction in SBP and a 1.93 mm Hg reduction in DBP in the CANVAS programme. Similar BP lowering has also been demonstrated by empagliflozin thus establishing an average 3–5 mm Hg SBP reduction by these drugs, which may offer an added benefit to most T2DM patients. A recent meta-analysis of RCTs and systematic review looking at the effects of SGLT-2 inhibitor on ambulatory BP showed significant reduction in 24-hour ambulatory systolic and diastolic BP by – 3.76 mm Hg (95% CI – 4.23 to – 2.34; I^2 = 0.99) and – 1.83 mm Hg (95% CI – 2.35 to – 1.31; I^2 = 0.76), respectively.

Owing to their BP lowering effects, there have been concerns of postural hypotension, dizziness and dehydration with these drugs in certain patients. These have been reported essentially in patients on loop diuretics and those with a glomerular filtration rate (GFR) <60 mL/min, more so in the elderly volume depleted patients, making it important to exercise caution in such patient groups.

Renal Effects—Acute Kidney Injury

Although there is sufficient data available from various landmark trials on the nephroprotection offered by SGLT-2 inhibitors in addition to their glycemic and CV benefits, there have been concerns on their use in patients with CKD. It is pertinent to understand that the SGLT-2 inhibitors work through the kidney, so the first consequence of renal impairment is reduced efficacy of these drugs in view of declining glomerular filtration. Hence current recommendations are for using these drugs in patients with an estimated GFR (eGFR) above 40 mL/min because of the lack of effectiveness at lower GFR rather than risks. The transient 2–4 mL/min fall in GFR seen with these agents in the first few weeks of initiation is a reversible phenomenon which eventually reverts back to baseline and does not deteriorate further. Hence in patients with T2DM with glomerular hyperfiltration, this actually may improve the GFR to normal levels possibly contributing to long-term nephroprotection.

The natriuresis and osmotic diuresis induced hypovolemia in addition to renal hemodynamic changes such as afferent arteriolar vasoconstriction as a result of restoration of impaired tubulo-glomerular feedback mechanism by increased drug-induced sodium delivery to the macula densa leading to adenosine release as well as increased glucagon levels may trigger an acute reversible GFR reduction. This reduction in intraglomerular pressure and reduced glomerular hyperfiltration has been shown in EMPA-REG, CANVAS as well as DECLARE trials to mediate long-term renal benefits, establishing their nephroprotective effects.

As the renin–angiotensin–aldosterone system (RAAS) blockers also offer similar short- and long-term renal protection, SGLT-2 inhibitors have emerged as another therapeutic option to provide additional renoprotection along with RAAS blockers in diabetic patients. However, the RAAS blockers also induce vasodilatation of the efferent arterioles. Hence concomitant administration of both the agents might induce an acute reduction in eGFR especially in patients with underlying extracellular volume depletion such as those on diuretics such as high dose furosemide, as well as those on agents altering renal hemodynamics such as NSAIDs. Concerns have been raised by the FDA and EMA about cases of acute kidney injury being reported making it important to be cautious when prescribing these agents in such patients. When used judiciously there is no additional risk of such events with these agents as shown in EMPA-REG, CANVAS as well as DECLARE trials where the rates of acute kidney injury in users versus non-users were almost similar or rather numerically lower.

HEMOCONCENTRATION AND STROKE

The SGLT-2 inhibitors induce diuresis, which may cause an increased hematocrit due to hemoconcentration, although other mechanisms such as increased eythropoietin levels leading to enhanced erythropoiesis have been proposed. This SGLT-2-induced hematocrit rise has been proposed to increase viscosity of blood, possibly increasing risk of stroke with this drug. This assumption was mainly based following a nonsignificant increase in stroke risk seen in the EMPA-REG OUTCOME trial (HR 1.18, 95% CI 0.89–1.56, p = 0.26 for fatal or nonfatal stroke; HR 1.24, 95% CI 0.92–1.67, p = 0.16 for nonfatal stroke). However these findings were not seen in both CANVAS (HR 0.87, 95% CI 0.69–1.09) as well as DECLARE (HR 1.01, 95% CI 0.84–1.21). Furthermore, a modified intent-to-treat analysis of the EMPA-REG OUTCOME study went on to reveal that the numeric increase in stroke seen in the empagliflozin arm was essentially due to a difference in patients with a first event more than 90 days after empagliflozin (18 patients in the empagliflozin arm vs. 3 in placebo arm) while there was no difference in incidence of stroke when events occurred while on treatment or ≤90 days after last dose of empagliflozin were analyzed (HR 1.08, 95% CI 0.81–1.45, p = 0.60). It is important to note that there was no increased stroke risk seen in patients who had the highest increments in hematocrit. Thus, though mechanistically SGLT-2 inhibitor induced hem concentration seems to be a culprit for increased strokes, a cause-effect etiology remains to be established in the current scenario with an inconclusive association between the two.

BONE EFFECTS AND FRACTURES

People with diabetes are known to have an increased risk of bone fractures, with T1DM being predisposed to increased risk for osteoporosis and an increased hip fracture incidence seen in those with T2DM. SGLT-2 inhibitor by virtue of their mechanism of action can potentially affect the renal tubular transport of bone minerals, making it pertinent to use these drugs with caution in patients who have an increased fracture risk. The osmotic diuresis induced by these drugs can cause volume depletion and dyselectrolytemia (serum calcium and phosphate). These agents increase serum phosphate concentrations which stimulate parathyroid hormone secretion and fibroblast growth factor 23 concentrations that may reduce vitamin D concentration and consequently calcium absorption. Increased parathyroid hormone increases bone resorption and on a background of reduced calcium absorption may reduce bone mineral density and increase risk of bone fractures, further potentiated by hyponatremia with these drugs.

This association was noticed in the CANVAS trial which set the alarm bells ringing (Table 2). Canagliflozin showed higher rates of fractures versus placebo (15.4 vs. 11.9 patients with fractures per 1,000 patient years; HR 1.26, CI 0.99–1.52). Heterogeneity in these findings was seen between the CANVAS and CANVAS-R studies in case of both low-trauma fractures as well as all fractures (both p ≤0.005) with CANVAS showing higher risk in the canagliflozin arm while CANVAS-R did not show such findings. Most of these were seen within a few weeks of taking the drug, were limited to upper extremities, and were more in subsets of older patients with a higher baseline CV risk, lower baseline eGFR and an increased diuretic usage; possibly ruling out bone-fragility as the culprit and suggesting falls on an outstretched arm especially in the elderly due to postural dizziness caused by volume depletion. Although this may primarily explain the mechanism of increased fracture risk, in another study canagliflozin administration has been associated with a decrease in total hip BMD (–0.9% and –1.2% with canagliflozin 100 mg and 300 mg respectively vs. placebo) over 204 weeks with no such decrease seen at other sites. In the same study, canagliflozin showed an increase in collagen type 1 beta-carboxy-telopeptide that correlated with a loss of body weight and an increase in osteocalcin, and a reduction in estradiol in women. Though empagliflozin also revealed few fracture incidences in T2DM patients with CKD in a double-blind RCT, no such signals were documented in the EMPA-REG OUTCOME trial. DECLARE-TIMI trial also did not show any such signal. Dapagliflozin did not show any effect on markers of bone formation and resorption as well as bone mineral density after 50 weeks of treatment in both male as well as postmenopausal females, thus negating any association with increased bone fractures risk with it. Few more recent meta-analyses have also revealed no increased bone fracture risk with SGLT-2 inhibitors. Nonetheless, caution may

TABLE 2: Effect of sodium-glucose linked transporter type 2 (SGLT-2) inhibitors on fracture risk.

STUDY (Type)	Sample size (n)	Agent used	Results
EMPA-REG OUTCOME (RCT)	7,020	Empagliflozin	With empagliflozin, there were no increased risk of fractures (3.9% in the placebo vs. 1.8% in the study group)
CANVAS (RCT)	10,142	Canagliflozin	As compared with placebo, there was increased fracture rate in the canagliflozin group (15.4 vs. 11.9 participants with fracture per 1,000 patient years HR 1.26, 95% CI 1.04–1.52)
Kohler et al. (Pooled analysis)	12,620	Empagliflozin	With empagliflozin, there were no increased risk of fractures (placebo 1.7%, empagliflozin 10 mg 1.6%, empagliflozin 25 mg 1.4% per 100 patient years)
Watts et al. (Pooled analysis)	10,194	Canagliflozin	With canagliflozin, there was increased risk of bone fractures (2.7% vs. 1.9% in the non-canagliflozin treatment group)
Tang et al. (Meta-analysis)	30,384	All SGLT-2 inhibitors	Both SGLT-2 inhibitors and placebo showed similar fracture risk (1.59% in the SGLT-2 inhibitor group vs. 1.56% in the placebo group)
			Similar event rates observed between all SGLT-2 inhibitors as compared with placebo (canagliflozin OR 1.15, 95% CI 0.71–1.88; dapagliflozin OR 0.68%, 95% CI 0.37–1.25 and empagliflozin OR 0.93, 95% CI 0.74–1.18)
Ruanpeng et al (Meta-analysis)	8,286	All SGLT-2 inhibitors	No increased fracture risk (RR 0.67 vs. placebo, 95% CI 0.42–1.07)
			Similar event rates observed between all SGLT-2 inhibitors as compared with placebo (RR for canagliflozin 0.66, 95% CI 0.37–1.19; RR for dapagliflozin 0.84, 95% CI 0.22–3.18 and RR for empagliflozin 0.57, 95% CI 0.20–1.59)

be exercised in using these agents in elderly osteoporotic patients till further conclusive evidences can be collected.

AMPUTATION RISK

Another important safety concern highlighted after the CANVAS trial is an increase in amputations mainly of the lower limbs—toes, feet and below legs, seen in patients on canagliflozin (6.3 vs. 3.5 per 1,000 patient years, p <0.001, HR 1.97, CI 1.41–2.75). About 715 of these amputations involved the toe or metatarsal, and was seen more in patients with prior peripheral vascular disease or those with a previous history of amputations. However both EMPA-REG OUTCOME study as well the DECLARE-TIMI did not corroborate this finding with amputation rates being similar in both groups. This lead to the conjecture that this was not essentially a class effect, though the exact cause could not be attributed to why it was specifically seen only with canagliflozin. Few cases of above-ankle or leg amputation also have been reported though the verdict is not yet out on its causation. Hence caution needs to be exercised in prescribing these drugs, primarily canagliflozin in such high-risk patients to avoid this morbid complication.

EFFECTS ON LIPIDS

Inspite of proving their CV benefits as well as safety, SGLT-2 inhibitors have been documented to cause a slight increase in low-density lipoprotein cholesterol (LDL-C). Patients with baseline LDL-C 90–110 mg/dL show a rise of about 5% with dapagliflozin 10 mg dose, 2.4% and 3.1% with empagliflozin 10 mg and 25 mg doses respectively and about 4–5% with canagliflozin 100 mg dose. Furthermore a slight increase in high-density lipoprotein cholesterol (HDL-C) to the tune of 6.8% and 6.1% with 100 mg and 300 mg doses of canagliflozin respectively as well as 6.3% with dapagliflozin 10 mg per day doses has been demonstrated. Though there has been talk of a counterbalancing of the detrimental effects of raised LDL-C with a concomitant increase in HDL-C, resulting in little or no change in the LDL-C/HDL-C ratio, it is a known fact that most HDL-C particles in patients with T2DM are dysfunctional, with markedly reduced antiatherogenic properties, thus offering hardly any cardioprotection with this rise. Though few studies have also demonstrated mild reduction in serum triglyceride levels, the long term effects of SGLT-2 inhibitors and their consequences are yet unknown.

SKIN DISORDERS

Few cases have been reported of drug eruptions 2–4 weeks after initiation of these drugs, described even as dehydration-related dyshidrotic eczema by dermatologists. A phase 3 RCT looking at ipragliflozin efficacy in Korean T2DM patients reported skin and subcutaneous tissue events in a very small fraction of patients. However, there near absence in the western world point towards a possible racial difference but this is yet to be established. All the three landmark SGLT-2 inhibitor trials did not report any significant skin effects with use of these drugs.

DRUG INTERACTIONS

Metabolism of canagliflozin has been found to be increased when used with UDP-glucuronosyltransferase (UGT) inducers such as rifampicin, phenobarbital, ritonavir and phenytoin, etc. resulting in reduced levels of active canagliflozin in blood, making it necessary to increase dose from 100 mg to 300 mg in such patients. Furthermore, canagliflozin has been shown to increase the area under the curve (AUC) for digoxin, hence these patients need regular monitoring when taking both. No major drug-drug interactions have been reported for dapagliflozin and empagliflozin.

CANCER RISK

The FDA Advisory Committee in 2011 raised concerns on malignancy risk on noting a non significant rise in number of breast and cancer reports in patients on dapagliflozin. By November 2013, there was evidence of 0.17% cases of bladder cancer (10 cases out of 6,045 users) in the dapagliflozin group versus just 0.03% (1 case among 3,512 individuals) in the placebo group. It is important to note that all 10 cases were reported within 2 years of drug initiation and 9 of these had documented hematuria within 6 months of starting the drug. Furthermore no fresh cases were reported between 2–4 years of drug exposure and these cases were quite heterogeneous ranging from invasive to non invasive and with variable grades, making a single etiology highly unlikely. Further, by 2013, there was also concern of increased breast cancer cases with dapagliflozin versus placebo with an incidence rate of 0.40 per 100 patient years (12 vs. 3 cases) in dapagliflozin group and 0.19 per 100 patient years in the placebo group. Again, all these were reported within 1 year of drug initiation and were heterogeneous in terms of age of the patients, tumor types, stages, etc. again ruling out a single causative trigger. These fears were laid to rest in the DECLARE-TIMI trial which reported much less cases of bladder cancer versus placebo [0.3% vs. 0.5%, HR 0.57 (0.35–0.93, p = 0.02)] as well as similar rates of breast cancer as placebo [0.4%, HR 1.02 (0.64–1.63, p = 0.92)]. Various other pooled analyses and meta-analyses failed to establish any significant causation with this drug. Similarly in CANVAS trial with canagliflozin bladder cancer and breast cancer rates did not significantly differ from the placebo group, showing no increased malignancy risk with the drug. In the EMPA-REG OUTCOME trial there was a significant increased bladder cancer rate reported in patients on empagliflozin (9 cases vs. none) but these were too low to establish a causation. Hence, though the association between SGLT-2 inhibitors and malignancy risk seems highly unlikely, these drugs may better be avoided in patients with hematuria or those at an increased cancer risk or previous history of bladder cancer till we have more long-term studies available.

CONCLUSION

The introduction of SGLT-2 inhibitors as a novel therapeutic option in the management of T2DM has ushered in a new era of changing paradigms based on a pathophysiology oriented treatment strategy. Besides proving their glycemic efficacy, these agents have fast gained acceptance globally owing to their pleiotropic benefits of weight loss, BP reduction and cardiorenal benefits. Apart from a slightly increased rate of genital and UTIs in predisposed patients, these are essentially well tolerated agents. As for malignancy concerns, except for the bladder cancer signal in dapagliflozin users that raised concerns, it seems highly unlikely to establish a causative association at this stage due to the early appearance of these signals with very less exposure time. Emphasis should be laid on avoiding these drugs in high-risk patients for these adverse events, such as those with recurrent or complicated UTIs and GTIs as well as those with hematuria or past history of bladder cancer. The need for regular follow-up with renal function monitoring is important to avoid untoward incidences of potential adverse effects. This once again highlights the need for careful selection of the right patient for these drugs to achieve maximum benefits.

SUGGESTED READING

1. American Diabetes Association. Standards of medical care in diabetes 2019. Diabetes Care. 2019;41(Suppl 1):S1-159.
2. Filippas-Ntekouan S, Filippatos TD, Elisaf MS. SGLT2 inhibitors: are they safe? Postgrad Med. 2018;130(1):72-82.
3. Kalra S, Ghosh S, Aamir AH, et al. Safe and pragmatic use of sodium–glucose co-transporter 2 inhibitors in type 2 diabetes mellitus: South Asian Federation of Endocrine Societies consensus statement. Indian J Endocrinol Metab. 2017;21(1):210.
4. Neal B, Perkovic V, Mahaffey KW, et al. Canagliflozin and cardiovascular and renal events in type 2 diabetes. The CANVAS Program Collaborative Group. N Engl J Med. 2017;377:644-57.
5. Rosenstock J, Ferrannini E. Euglycemic Diabetic Ketoacidosis: A Predictable, Detectable, and Preventable Safety Concern With SGLT2 Inhibitors Diabetes Care. 2015;38(9):1638-42.
6. Rosenstock J, Seman LJ, Jelaska A, et al. Efficacy and safety of empagliflozin, a sodium glucose cotransporter 2 (SGLT-2) inhibitor, as add-on to metformin in type 2 diabetes with mild hyperglycemia. Diabetes Obes Metab. 2013;15:1154-60.
7. Singh AK, Unnikrishnan AG, Zargar AH, et al. Evidence-Based Consensus on Positioning of SGLT2 iin Type 2 Diabetes Mellitus in Indians. Diabetes Ther. 2019.
8. Singh M, Kumar A. Risks Associated with SGLT2 Inhibitors: An Overview. Curr Drug Saf. 2018;13(2):84-91.
9. Tsimihodimos V, Filippatos TD, Elisaf MS. Effects of sodium-glucose cotransporter 2 inhibitors on metabolism: unanswered questions and controversies. Expert Opin Drug MetabToxicol. 2017;13:399-408.
10. Ueda P, Svanström H, Melbye M, et al. Sodium glucose cotransporter 2 inhibitors and risk of serious adverse events: nationwide register based cohort study. BMJ. 2018;363:k4365.
11. Wiviott SD, Raz I, Bonaca MP, et al. Dapagliflozin and Cardiovascular Outcomes in Type 2 Diabetes. The DECLARE-TIMI 58 investigators. N Engl J Med. 2019;380:347-57.
12. Zinman B, Wanner C, Lachin JM, et al. Empagliflozin, Cardiovascular Outcomes, and Mortality in Type 2 Diabetes. The EMPAREG OUTCOME Investigators. N Engl J Med. 2015;373:2117-28.

7
CHAPTER

SGLT-2 Inhibitors in Diabetes: Place in Management Algorithms

INTRODUCTION

The management of diabetes has undergone a sea change in recent times with focus shifting from a glucocentric approach to a holistic patient-centered pathophysiology-based management strategy aimed at not only tackling glucotoxicity and relieving symptoms of acute hyperglycemia but also establishing a stable glucose control with minimal glycemic variability to achieve the long-term goals of preventing/delaying complications, effective cardiovascular risk management, and restoring a better quality of life for these patients. A strategy that preserves β-cell function and slows the rate of β-cell apoptosis to delay the natural progression of diabetes can be utopia for a patient with type 2 diabetes (T2D). All guidelines stress upon individualized management for each patient. Lifestyle management including increased physical activity aimed at weight loss especially in overweight/obese individuals and a healthy diet guided by medical nutrition therapy along with smoking cessation and psychological support form the mainstay of therapy in all guidelines and consensus statements. Atherosclerotic cardiovascular disease (ASCVD) has been recognized as a leading cause of death in type 2 diabetes mellitus (T2DM) and it is well established that diabetes itself confers a substantial ASCVD risk, thus highlighting the importance of controlling the modifiable ASCVD risk factors in these patients to reduce this risk as it has been demonstrated in various studies. This brings us to the concept of multifactorial management of T2DM where use of pharmacotherapy with both oral as well as injectable agents in addition to lifestyle modification strategies as mentioned earlier is recommended to achieve the glycated hemoglobin target of less than 7% in order to prevent complications.

As discussed in earlier chapters, the two main sodium-glucose cotransporters (SGLTs)—SGLT-1 and SGLT-2 have emerged as new therapeutic agents in our armamentarium to manage type 2 diabetes. SGLT-1, active primarily in the small intestine and the SGLT-2, predominant in the kidneys both reabsorb glucose back into circulation contributing to worsening hyperglycemia and T2D. Inhibitors of these transporters with varying specificities for each of them (e.g. empagliflozin, dapagliflozin, canagliflozin, etc.) work by reducing intestinal as well as renal glucose reabsorption and increasing urinary excretion of excess glucose from the body, thus contributing to not only reduced hyperglycemia but also weight loss and blood pressure reduction and cardiorenal benefits. Randomized clinical trials as well as real-world studies have established their glucose-lowering efficacy and sustained action when used as monotherapy as well as add-on therapy to other agents including insulin. Increased urinary glucose excretion may predispose to a higher risk of urinary and genital infections while excessive SGLT-1 inhibition may cause gastrointestinal symptoms. This underlines the need to use these agents in a correctly selected patient based on his individual profile. Their insulin-independent mechanism of action offers durable glycemic control with minimum hypoglycemia at any stage of T2D along its natural history. New data is emerging fast on their efficacy in type 1 diabetes in addition to insulin and may eventually establish them in the future as novel agents in this group of patients as well.

POSITIONING OF SGLT-2 INHIBITORS IN THERAPY

The choice of agents for management of T2DM involves due consideration of not only the efficacy, tolerability and safety of the agent but also durability of its action. Other factors such as patient preference and cost, glycemic targets, polypharmacy, comorbidities, and side effect profile also play a very important role in choosing the best agent. Besides, the new 2018 American Diabetes Association (ADA)-European Association for the Study of

Diabetes (EASD) Consensus Statement on management of T2DM gives extreme importance to considering a history of CVD very early when selecting glucose-lowering agent for patients with T2DM. The emerging evidence on favorable effects of specific medications [SGLT-2 inhibitors as well as glucagon-like peptide-1 (GLP-1) receptor agonists] in reducing mortality, heart failure (HF), and progression of renal disease in patients with established CVD compel their preferential use in this particular group. Further, SGLT-2 inhibitors are recommended in ASCVD patients with coexisting HF or concerns of HF owing to their proven benefits in such patients. The renal benefits in terms of reduced chronic kidney disease (CKD) progression with use of SGLT-2 inhibitors have also placed them as recommended agents in T2DM with CKD progression.

The progressive nature of T2D, characterized by gradual loss of β-cell function manifested as declining insulin secretion, is deemed responsible for secondary failure of various agents such as sulfonylureas with time. The insulin-independent action of SGLT-2 inhibitors, thus, places these novel agents as an efficacious option across all stages in the natural history of disease provided the renal function is adequate and patient is adequately insulinized (exogenous or endogenous). By increasing urinary glucose excretion, these agents counter glucotoxicity, thereby reducing insulin resistance and β-cell damage leading to an improved metabolic milieu in the body by restoring euglycemia.

Use of SGLT-2 inhibitors as monotherapy as well as add-on to other agents have demonstrated glucose-lowering efficacy of these agents in patients with T2D. They can be used effectively after metformin. They may be especially useful in overweight/obese T2DM patients especially in those where obesity-related comorbid issues such as sleep apnea or hypertension further reduce their quality of life. Monotherapy with these agents may be considered in patients intolerant to metformin, but with adequate renal function. As these drugs work primarily through the kidneys, efficacy of these drugs is reduced in renal impairment and hence currently they are not indicated for use in patients with estimated glomerular filtration rate (eGFR) <45 mL/min/1.73 m^2 (though studies have shown their safety at an eGFR of even 30 mL/min/1.73 m^2).

In patients with concerns of hypoglycemia, a reduction in dose of a sulfonylurea or insulin is recommended when initiating an SGLT-2 inhibitor. As an add-on to insulin, SGLT-2 inhibitors reduce insulin dose requirement and offset the insulin-induced weight gain. These drugs can even be used as part of a triple drug regimen in uncontrolled type 2 diabetics with preserved renal function with or without insulin. Though these drugs have shown safety in the elderly, but in patients older than 75 years, their use is restricted as efficacy is compromised with decreasing renal function and may also cause postural hypotension and dizziness. Though renal impairment is a common complication of diabetes, there is no evidence of renal damage with these agents. The osmotic diuresis induced by these agents may cause a little reduction in extracellular volume akin to initiation of diuretic therapy, causing a temporary reduction in GFR which eventually stabilizes back without causing any major renal insult. Caution also needs to be exercised when using these agents with a loop diuretic owing to their potential effects on sodium excretion.

Sodium-glucose cotransporter-2 inhibitors have been recommended much higher up as preferential agents not only by the ADA-EASD 2018 Consensus Statement, even the American Association of Clinical Endocrinologists (AACE)/American College of Endocrinology (ACE) Guidelines 2018 also recommend these novel agents in their algorithm for T2DM management much higher up in hierarchy than other agents. These guidelines recommend initiation of monotherapy with metformin for all T2DM patients followed by GLP-1 receptor agonists, SGLT-2 inhibitors, dipeptidyl peptidase-4 inhibitor (DPP-4 inhibitor), and then thiazolidinediones (TZDs) in the corresponding order of hierarchy followed by α-glucosidase inhibitors and by sulfonylureas when the hemoglobin A1c (HbA1c) is less than 7.5%. When commencing dual therapy at HbA1c >7.5% or triple therapy at HbA1c >9% for initiation in T2D patients with no osmotic symptoms, these guidelines place these agents at top of the hierarchy giving their order of preference based not only on their glycemic efficacy but also less incidence of hypoglycemia and pleiotropic benefits of reduction in blood pressure and body weight as well as cardiorenal benefits.

The ADA-EASD approach is essentially based on assessment of key characteristics such as current lifestyle, comorbidities (ASCVD, CKD, HF), clinical profile of the patient (age, weight, HbA1c at presentation, etc.), clinical as well as socioeconomic status, and issues such as motivation, depression, etc. The choice of the agent involves due consideration of specific factors such as target HbA1c, impact of the agent on hypoglycemia, body weight, its side effect profile, cost, access, and availability which ensure adherence to therapy. The recommended management strategy involves shared decision making by both the patient and the prescriber to formulate and implement an individualized management plan tailor-made for each individual patient that can be reviewed from time to time and modified as per the needs to ensure efficacy of the plan while avoiding clinical inertia in decision making to achieve the target glycemic control at goal and prevent complications while optimizing the quality of life of the individual patient.

The AACE/ACE comprehensive T2DM management algorithm adopts a slightly different approach wherein it suggests agent choices based on the HbA1c at presentation and places the available agents in a hierarchy based on their different characteristics. So, the choice of agent as monotherapy, dual, or even triple therapy is based on presenting symptoms as well as HbA1c at presentation and multiple agents can then be added-on one after the other as per their placement in the hierarchy. The order of preference places metformin as the first agent of choice for monotherapy and any other agent only if metformin is not tolerated or contraindicated. The order of preference varies slightly with GLP-1 receptor agonists, SGLT-2 inhibitors, and DPP-4 inhibitors followed by TZD and basal insulin for dual therapy, while for triple therapy DPP-4 inhibitors are placed lower down after TZD and basal insulin. It is important to note that AACE/ACE algorithm places sulfonylureas much lower down in the hierarchy because of their propensity to cause significant adverse effects like hypoglycemia and weight gain (Flowchart 1).

The AACE/ACE guidelines just like the ADA-EASD guidelines acknowledge the benefits of SGLT-2 inhibitors in T2DM patients especially the ones with ASCVD and hence accord them a preferred position higher up early on in therapy owing to not only their glycemic efficacy but also their blood pressure (BP) lowering and weight loss effects contributing to cardiorenal pleiotropic benefits. Correct patient choice is of extreme importance when choosing these agents and hence these agents can safely be used in all T2DM patients who have suboptimal control, are overweight or obese, have optimum renal function (up to an eGFR of 45 mL/min/1.73 m^2), and are not insulin deficient. These agents can be used in combination with all other available antidiabetic agents including insulin based on individual patient profiles and are efficacious in all stages in the natural progression of diabetes. The benefits of BP reduction and weight loss in addition to reduced propensity for hypoglycemia and durability of action make them preferred agents in the current armamentarium of antidiabetic drugs available to us.

CONCLUSION

The ADA-EASD 2018 Consensus Statement as well as the AACE/ACE 2018 Algorithm for management of T2DM is based on two different approaches to reach target glycemic control for each patient based on his individual profile and needs. In this era of evidence-based precision medicine, there is no one size fits all management strategy and treatment has to tailor-made for each individual patient involving a carefully formulated management plan. By decreasing renal glucose reabsorption and increasing urinary glucose excretion, SGLT-2 inhibitors have emerged as novel antihyperglycemic agents that can reduce hyperglycemia in an insulin-independent manner working all stages of T2DM besides the added benefits of weight loss and blood pressure control. Slight inhibition of SGLT-1 can further delay intestinal glucose absorption, although these effects are not potent enough to cause hypoglycemia or transfer of glucose into the large intestine. Glucosuria does aggravate concerns of genital and urinary tract infections in a very small percentage of patients but proper patient education and preventive measures can avoid these, and overall tolerability has been good with these agents. Meticulously conducted randomized clinical trials followed by real-world studies and experiences have consistently confirmed the efficacy of these agents as monotherapy as well as add-on therapy to all other glucose-lowering agents including insulin in a correctly chosen patient. The cardiorenal benefits observed in patients with T2DM with established ASCVD have led to their recommendation

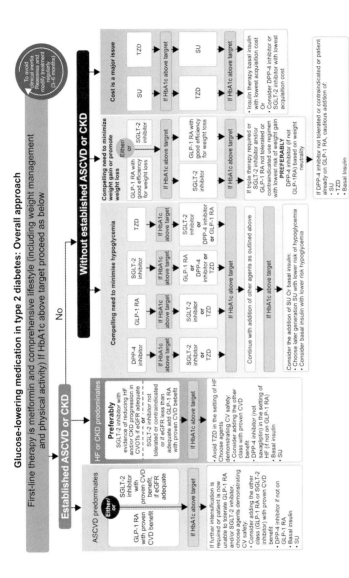

(ASCVD: atherosclerotic cardiovascular disease; CKD: chronic kidney disease; CVOTs: Cardiovascular Outcome Trials; DPP-4: dipeptidyl peptidase-4; eGFR: estimated glomerular filtration rate; GLP-1 RA: glucagon-like peptide-1 receptor agonist; HbA1c: hemoglobin A1c; HF: heart failure; SGLT-2: sodium-glucose cotransporter-2; TZD: thiazolidinediones)

FLOWCHART 1: Glucose-lowering medication in type 2 diabetes: Overall approach.

Source: Pharmacologic Approaches to Glycemic Treatment: Standards of Medical Care in Diabetes 2019. American Diabetes Association. Diabetes Care. 2019;42(Suppl. 1):S90-S102.

as preferred agents all across the world in this group giving them a much coveted slot right at the top of all treatment algorithms for T2DM.

SUGGESTED READING

1. American Diabetes Association. 9. Cardiovascular Disease and Risk Management: Standards of Medical Care in Diabetes-2018. Diabetes Care. 2018;41(Suppl 1):S86-104.

2. Bailey CJ. The challenge of managing coexistent type 2 diabetes and obesity. BMJ. 2011;342:d1996.

3. Barnett AH, Ali O, Bailey CJ, et al. Recommendations regarding the position of dapagliflozin within the type 2 diabetes treatment algorithm. Diabetes Prac. 2013;2(2):1-11.

4. Buse JB, Bergenstal RM, Glass LC, et al. Use of twice-daily exenatide in basal insulin-treated patients with type 2 diabetes: a randomized, controlled trial. Ann Intern Med. 2011;154(2):103-12.

5. Dapagliflozin (Forxiga). (2012). Summary of Product Characteristics. [online] Available from http://www. medicines.org.uk/EMC/medicine/27188/. [Accessed January, 2019].

6. Davies MJ, D'Alessio DA, Fradkin J, et al. Management of hyperglycaemia in type 2 diabetes, 2018. A consensus report by the American Diabetes Association (ADA) and the European Association for the Study of Diabetes (EASD). Diabetologia. 2018;61(12):2461-98.

7. DeFronzo RA, Davidson JA, Del Prato S. The role of the kidneys in glucose homeostasis: a new path towards normalizing glycaemia. Diabetes Obes Metab. 2012;14(1):5-14.

8. DeFronzo RA. From the Triumvirate to the Ominous Octet: A New Paradigm for the Treatment of Type 2 Diabetes Mellitus. Diabetes. 2009;58(4):773-95.

9. Ferrannini E, Solini A. SGLT2 inhibition in diabetes mellitus: rationale and clinical prospects. Nat Rev Endocrinol. 2012;8(8):495-502.

10. Foote C, Perkovic V, Neal B. Effects of SGLT2 inhibitors on cardiovascular outcomes. Diab Vasc Dis Res. 2012;9(2):117-23.

11. Gerich JE, Meyer C, Woerle HJ, et al. Renal gluconeogenesis: its importance in human glucose homeostasis. Diabetes Care. 2001;24(2):382-91.

12. Handelsman Y, Bloomgarden ZT, Grunberger G, et al. American Association of Clinical Endocrinologists and American College of Endocrinology—clinical practice guidelines for developing a diabetes mellitus comprehensive care plan—2015. Endocr Pract. 2015;21 (Suppl 1):1-87.

13. Lee YJ, Lee YJ, Han HJ. Regulatory mechanisms of Na(+)/glucose cotransporters in renal proximal tubule cells. Kidney Int Suppl. 2007;106:S27-35.

14. Nauck MA, Del Prato S, Meier JJ, et al. Dapagliflozin versus glipizide as add-on therapy in patients with type 2 diabetes who have inadequate glycemic control with

metformin: a randomized, 52-week, double-blind, active-controlled noninferiority trial. Diabetes Care. 2011;34(9):2015-22.

15. Seman L, Macha S, Nehmiz G, et al. Empagliflozin (BI 10773), a potent and selective SGLT2 inhibitor, induces dose-dependent glucosuria in healthy subjects. Clin Pharmacol Drug Dev. 2013;2(2):152-61.

16. Sha S, Devineni D, Ghosh A, et al. Canagliflozin, a novel inhibitor of sodium glucose co-transporter 2, dose dependently reduces the calculated renal threshold for glucose excretion and increases urinary glucose excretion in healthy subjects. Diabetes Obes Metab. 2011;13(7):669-72.

17. Shirazi-Beechey SP, Moran AW, Batchelor DJ, et al. Glucose sensing and signalling; regulation of intestinal glucose transport. Proc Nutr Soc. 2011;70(2):185-93.

18. Stümpel F, Burcelin R, Jungermann K, et al. Normal kinetics of intestinal glucose absorption in the absence of GLUT2: evidence for a transport pathway requiring glucose phosphorylation and transfer into the endoplasmic reticulum. Proc Natl Acad Sci. 2001;98(20):11330-5.

19. Tahrani AA, Bailey CJ, Del Prato S, et al. Management of type 2 diabetes: new and future developments in treatment. Lancet. 2011;378(9786):182-97.

8

CHAPTER

Clinical Pearls: Indications, Contraindications and Caution in Use of SGLT-2 Inhibitors

INTRODUCTION

Sodium-glucose cotransporter 2 (SGLT-2) inhibitors have a unique mechanism of action and lead to glycemic reduction independent of insulin action. Owing to their extra glycemic benefits, SGLT-2 inhibitors have become an important therapeutic option in the treatment of diabetes especially in patients not willing to start insulin. SGLT-2 inhibitors may also be an excellent option in patients with high cardiovascular risk profile and in obese and hypertensive patients because of their potential weight loss and antihypertensive benefits. Patients at high risk of hypoglycemia will benefit from a combination of SGLT-2 inhibitor and metformin as risk of hypoglycemia with SGLT-2 inhibitors is minimal as compared to sulfonylureas (SUs) or insulin. Moreover, SGLT-2 inhibitors are equally effective across the spectrum of disease as their action is independent of β-cell function and insulin secretion. SGLT-2 inhibitors remains equally effective even in long-standing diabetes as long as renal function is adequate.

CLINICAL BENEFICIAL EFFECTS

- SGLT-2 inhibitors lead to significant fasting and postprandial glucose reduction—not many oral antidiabetic drugs decrease both together (See Table 1 comparing HbA1c reduction of all oral antidiabetic agents)
- *Lower hypoglycemia risk*: As SGLT-2 inhibitors do not stimulate pancreatic β-cells and insulin secretion, there is no risk of hypo-

glycemia as compared to other medications, particularly SUs and insulin. However, in combination with SUs and insulin risk of hypoglycemia increases
- *Significant weight loss*: SGLT-2 inhibitors lead to a 3–4 kg weight reduction as compared to placebo
- *Systolic blood pressure reduction*: Osmotic diuresis and Natriuresis as a result of action on the renal tubules leads to systolic blood pressure reduction by 3–5 mm Hg
- Cardio renal benefits as explained earlier.

CAUTION

- Mycotic infections and vulvovaginal candidiasis were most common side effects seen approximately in 10% females in phase 3 clinical trials
- Osmotic diuresis reduces intravascular volume and leads to orthostatic hypotension. Renal glycosuria drugs water and solute with it causing dehydration as well
- Diuresis leads to hyperkalemia and renal insufficiency. It is recommended that KFT should be checked in 2 week's time after starting SGLT-2 inhibitors and regularly thereafter
- SGLT-2 inhibitors dosages must be titrated based on estimated glomerular filtration rate (eGFR) as suggested in Table 2

TABLE 1: HbA1c reduction comparison with various oral antidiabetic medications.

Oral antidiabetic medications	HbA1c reduction (%)*
SGLT-2 inhibitors	0.7–1.0
Biguanides	1.0–1.5
Sulfonylureas	1.0–1.5
Meglitinides	0.5–1.0
Dipeptidyl peptidase 4 inhibitors	0.5–1.0
Thiazolidinediones	1.0–1.5
Alpha-glucosidase inhibitors	0.5–1.0

*The HbA1c reduction is based on data reported in clinical trials and may be influenced by baseline HbA1c, duration and severity of disease (β-cell function remaining), and drug's mechanism of action. HbA1c lowering effect may differ in each patient.

(HbA1c: glycated hemoglobin)

TABLE 2: SGLT-2 inhibitor dosage adjustments based on renal function.

eGFR mL/min/1.73 m^2	Empagliflozin	Canagliflozin	Dapagliflozin
≥60	No dosage adjustment 10–25 mg /day	No dosage adjustment 100–300 mg/day	No dosage adjustment 5–10 mg/day
45–60	10 mg daily	100 mg daily	Not recommended eGFR <60
30–45	Not recommended	Not recommended eGFR <45	N/A
<30	Contra-indicated	Contraindicated	Contraindicated

(SGTL-2: sodium-glucose cotransporter 2)

- SGLT-2 inhibitors are quite expensive as of now so cost-benefit must be assessed along with patient's affordability
- SGLT-2 inhibitors may increase low-density lipoprotein (LDL) cholesterol by 2 to 3%, though the exact mechanism responsible is not known. CVOTs with SGLT-2 inhibitors have proved that these drugs are effective at reducing cardiovascular events. So this small increase in LDL may not mean much
- SGLT-2 inhibitors are contraindicated in patients with renal insufficiency [glomerular filtration rate (GFR) <45 mL/min/1.73 m^2]
- Patients with history of hematuria or bladder malignancy must not be prescribed these agents
- Canagliflozin has been shown to cause a slight increase in lower limb amputations primarily of toes, more so in patients with peripheral vascular disease (PVD) or prior history of diabetic foot ulcers, hence caution may be exercised in prescribing these agents in such patients till further clarity is obtained.

CLINICAL PEARLS

- SGLT-2 inhibitors have a novel mechanism of preventing glucose reabsorption from proximal convoluted tubule (PCT) producing glycosuria and subsequent glycemic reduction without stimulating insulin release
- SGLT-2 inhibitors work independent of β-cell function and insulin secretion, thus can be very useful in patients with long-standing diabetes with preserved renal function

- SGLT-2 inhibitors have demonstrated noninferiority along with added metabolic benefits of sustained weight loss and blood pressure reduction
- The renal glycosuria has the potential to increase fungal growth especially in the genitourinary tract and perineum, predisposing the patients to increased risk for genital mycotic infections. Although in clinical trials as well as real world studies genital mycotic infections, urinary tract infections and osmotic diuresis related adverse events have been reported, these were normally mild to moderate in intensity and generally treatable by standard course of antibiotics/antifungals and did not recur, hence in most cases drug discontinuation is not required
- There is an increase in the risk of diabetic ketoacidosis with SGLT-2 inhibitors on a background of uncharacteristically mild-to-moderate glucose elevations [euglycemic diabetic ketoacidosis (DKA)]. Though FDA did acknowledge that most cases did occur where the drug was used off-label in type 1 diabetes mellitus (T1DM) patients, yet its occurrence in type 2 diabetes mellitus (T2DM) patients has been documented. T2DM who developed this complication were mostly hospitalized patients in a catabolic state or with severe sepsis, indicating that we need to be careful about when prescribing this drug in these type of patients

Flowchart 1 shows the proposed algorithm for adjusting anti-diabetic/antihypertensive agent's doses when starting SGLT-2 inhibitor therapy.

- Under titrate diuretic/antihypertensive therapy—ensure that patient is hemodynamically stable lest there is orthostatic hypo-tension or blood pressure liability or syncope etc.
- When initiating SGLT-2 inhibitors in patients with type 2 diabetes already on high doses of SUs—reduce the doses of SUs to prevent hypoglycemia as shown in the algorithm below
- Avoid immediate insulin withdrawal to minimize the risk of euglycemic DKA. Subsequently adjust insulin doses once glucose levels start falling. Ensure an adequate carbohydrate intake as well to prevent ketosis
- Ensure enough oral fluid intake to prevent dehydration and postural hypotension especially in elderly patients.

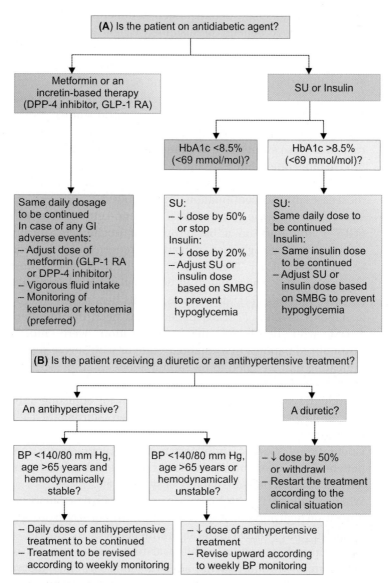

(A) Is the patient on antidiabetic agent?

Metformin or an incretin-based therapy (DPP-4 inhibitor, GLP-1 RA)

SU or Insulin

HbA1c <8.5% (<69 mmol/mol)?

HbA1c >8.5% (<69 mmol/mol)?

Same daily dosage to be continued
In case of any GI adverse events:
– Adjust dose of metformin (GLP-1 RA or DPP-4 inhibitor)
– Vigorous fluid intake
– Monitoring of ketonuria or ketonemia (preferred)

SU:
– ↓ dose by 50% or stop
Insulin:
– ↓ dose by 20%
– Adjust SU or insulin dose based on SMBG to prevent hypoglycemia

SU:
Same daily dose to be continued
Insulin:
– Same insulin dose to be continued
– Adjust SU or insulin dose based on SMBG to prevent hypoglycemia

(B) Is the patient receiving a diuretic or an antihypertensive treatment?

An antihypertensive?

A diuretic?

BP <140/80 mm Hg, age >65 years and hemodynamically stable?

BP <140/80 mm Hg, age >65 years or hemodynamically unstable?

– ↓ dose by 50% or withdrawl
– Restart the treatment according to the clinical situation

– Daily dose of antihypertensive treatment to be continued
– Treatment to be revised according to weekly monitoring

– ↓ dose of antihypertensive treatment
– Revise upward according to weekly BP monitoring

(BP: blood pressure; DPP-4: dipeptidyl peptidase-4; GI: gastrointestinal; GLP-1 RA: glucagon-like peptide-1 receptor agonist; HbA1c: glycated hemoglobin; SU: sulfonylureas)

FLOWCHART 1: Proposed algorithm for adjusting antidiabetic/antihypertensive agent's doses when starting SGLT-2 inhibitor therapy.

CONCLUSION

The SGLT-2 inhibitors are novel agents having a unique mechanism to treat patients with type 2 diabetes throughout the natural history of the disease due to their β-cell independent action. SGLT-2 inhibitors are fast emerging as efficacious agents for management of type 2 diabetes with their pleiotropic benefits like weight loss, blood pressure reduction as well as cardiovascular and renal benefits. These agents are increasingly being used as adjunct therapy for type 1 diabetes under strict physician supervision. As a result their acceptability as antidiabetic drugs is fast improving and most guidelines today place them much higher in the hierarchy as choice of preferred agents for diabetes control. Though these drugs have multiple benefits, they do come with their own share of side effects and safety issues that one has to be vigilant about. The most frequently reported adverse events such as euglycemic diabetic ketoacidosis, urinary tract infections, genital mycotic infections etc. have been reported as a class effect with these agents.

SUGGESTED READING

1. Desouza CV, Gupta N, Patel A. Cardiometabolic Effects of a New Class of Antidiabetic Agents. ClinTher.2015;37(6):1178-94.
2. Farxiga® [package insert]. Princeton, NJ: Bristol-Myers Squibb; 2014.
3. Handelsman Y, Henry RR, Bloomgarden ZT, et al. American Association of Clinical Endocrinologists and American College of Endocrinology position statement on the association of SGLT-2 inhibitors and diabetic ketoacidosis. Endocr Pract. 2016;22:753-62.
4. Invokana®[package insert]. Titusville, NJ: Janssen Pharmaceuticals, Inc; 2013.
5. Inzucchi SE, Bergenstal RM, Buse JB, et al. Management of hyperglycemia in type 2 diabetes: a patient-centered approach: position statement of the American Diabetes Association (ADA) and the European Association for the Study of Diabetes (EASD). Diabetes Care. 2012;35:1364-79.
6. Nathan DM, Buse JB, Davidson MB, et al. Medical management of hyperglycemia in type 2 diabetes: a consensus algorithm for the initiation and adjustment of therapy: a consensus statement of the American Diabetes Association and the European Association for the Study of Diabetes. Diabetes Care. 2009;32:193-203.
7. Stenlof K, Cefalu WT, Kim KA, et al. Efficacy and safety of canagliflozin monotherapy in subjects with type 2 diabetes mellitus inadequately controlled with diet and exercise. Diabetes Obes Metab. 2013;15:373-82.

SGLT-2 Inhibitors in Type 1 Diabetes: Emerging Evidences

INTRODUCTION

Type 1 diabetes mellitus (T1DM) is a state of absolute insulin deficiency caused by an autoimmune (or idiopathic in 20% cases) destruction of the β-cells of the pancreas necessitating a lifelong need for insulin for glycemic control and survival. Much to our chagrin, in spite of so many advancements in insulin development and delivery, a large number of patients are still not on target control, and this leads to similar micro- as well as macrovascular complications of diabetes as in type 2 diabetes mellitus (T2DM), albeit at earlier ages in patients with T1DM. Data from studies such as DCCT as well as EDIC have clearly shown that not only the poor metabolic memory contributes to this, but also their long term data clearly highlight the benefits of early and intensive glycemic control in reducing risk of these complications. Furthermore, there is a rising trend of obesity and weight gain seen in patients with T1DM, giving rise to a mixed diabetes like picture where the T1DM patient shows additional features of insulin resistance like in T2DM secondary to weight gain. The pediatric diabetes consortium and the SEARCH for Diabetes in Youth Study pegged the prevalence of overweight and obesity amongst newly diagnosed T1DM individuals at 21–22%, attributed to the global obesity epidemic worsened by sedentarism, family history as well as ethnic predisposition to obesity among other factors. Thus there has been a search for non-insulin adjunctive therapies that can not only aid insulin in achieving better glycemic control, but also minimize weight gain with reduced insulin doses and reduce complications as well as offer cardiovascular and renal benefits or protection. Although there have been reports of various agents such as metformin, pioglitazone, pramlintide, glucagon-like peptide-1 receptor agonists (GLP-1 RAs), SGLT-2 inhibitors as well as dual SGLT-1–SGLT-2 inhibitors being studied as potential adjunctive non-insulin therapies in T1DM, their success has been limited and there is need for more data supporting their use before they can be recommended for use in T1DM patients in addition to insulin.

NEED FOR ADJUVANT THERAPIES IN T1DM

The discovery of Insulin was a historical landmark in the management of T1DM, bringing forth a new ray of life into what was otherwise doomed as a death sentence with zero survival rates for such individuals. We have travelled a long distance from injecting coarse animal extracts to designer insulins and novel drug delivery technologies ranging from insulin pumps to even bionic pancreas soon becoming a reality. Unfortunately, in spite of this, not more than 20% of our diabetic patients are in target HbA1c less than 7%. To make matters worse, 40–50% of T1DM patients now also have features of metabolic syndrome including obesity and need higher and higher doses of insulin for better control, resulting in increased risk of hypoglycemia as well as weight gain. Thus there is a definite need for add-on therapies to insulin for these patients which can not only help achieve target glycemic control but also offer added benefits of weight loss and reduced insulin doses. There have been various molecules that have been documented as probable adjuvant candidates, most important being metformin, glitazones, pramlintide as well as GLP-1 RAs. With the advent of SGLT-2 inhibitors as novel drugs working through an insulin independent mechanism, they offer a new hope in this segment, more so with their BP and weight reducing potential and cardiorenal benefits. A lot of data is fast emerging on this yet "off-label" use of these agents and maybe these drugs could one day be recommended as adjuvant therapy for T2DM patients if they successfully stand the test of time. The concern of their ketogenic potential is real and this mandates detailed studies in this area as well as cautious prescription of these drugs in T1DM patients with careful titration of insulin doses.

CURRENT EVIDENCES

Different SGLT-2 inhibitors from this class of drugs have been tried in T1DM patients across the globe in well controlled studies. Several short-duration prospective, randomized pilot studies involving remogliflozin, dapagliflozin and empagliflozin demonstrated significant glycemic reductions with improved HbA1c, paving the way for future long term studies with larger patient populations to explore their use in T1DM. An increase of 72–88 g/24 h. in urinary glucose excretion was documented with dapagliflozin in 70 adults with T1DM along with an insulin dose reduction of 16.2–19.3%, significant reduction in 24-hour average glucose and glycemic variability without any major safety concerns in the two-week study period. Another 24-week study with dapagliflozin also demonstrated significant reductions in fasting as well as postprandial blood glucose levels, HbA1c, total cholesterol, LDL cholesterol and triglycerides in T1DM subjects. Another study showed similar results when dapagliflozin was added to T1DM subjects as add-on therapy to insulin and liraglutide.

Empagliflozin as an add-on to Insulin in 75 T1DM individuals showed significant increase in 24-hour urinary glucose excretion along with an HbA1c reduction of –0.35 to –0.49% and a total daily insulin dose reduction by –0.07 to –0.09 U/kg and weight loss of –1.5 to –1.9 kg, without any significant increase in hypoglycemia rates. A significant reduction in area under curve for 24-hour mean glucose was seen in the empagliflozin subjects, showing an adjusted mean difference of –30.2 mg/dL/h (95% CI –42.2 to –18.2) with empagliflozin 10 mg daily dose and –33.0 mg/dL/h (95% CI –44.8 to –21.1) with empagliflozin 25 mg dose. There was a significant reduction in glycemic variability with an increased time spent in target glucose range without any significant increase in hypoglycemia events.

Another small study using triple combination therapy of insulin, liraglutide and dapagliflozin in T1DM patients showed improved glycemic control with an HbA1c reduction of 0.66%, an increase in percent time spent in the glycemic range of 70–160 mg/dL of 11%, a decrease in >160 mg/dL of 13% and a 2-kg weight loss over 12 weeks. These improvements were seen over and above those attained with insulin and liraglutide, though one patient did develop diabetic ketoacidosis (DKA) in spite of normal glucose levels. A study with sotagliflozin, a dual SGLT-1 and SGLT-2 inhibitor also demonstrated similar results with an HbA1c reduction of 0.55%, reduced doses of bolus insulin doses, 1.7 kg weight reduction and a 14% increase in time spent in target glucose range of 70–180 mg/dL and a reduction in time spent in hyperglycemic range >180 mg/dL.

A meta-analysis by Yang et al. on use of SGLT-2 inhibitors in T1DM found an absolute reduction in fasting blood glucose [mean differences (MD) -2.47 mmol/L, 95% confidence interval (CI) -3.65 to -1.28, p <0.001] and insulin dosage (standardized MD -0.75 U, 95% CI -1.17 to -0.33, p <0.001) along with an increased urinary glucose reduction (MD 131.09 g/day; p <0.001). There was no significant increase in incidence rates of urinary or genital tract infections and diabetic ketoacidosis, with the authors commenting that SGLT-2 inhibitors may be an efficient and safe treatment option for patients with T1DM as an add-on drug with insulin.

The dapagliflozin evaluation in patients with inadequately controlled Type 1 diabetes (DEPICT-1) was a double-blind, randomized, parallel-controlled, three-arm, phase 3, multicenter study done at 143 sites in 17 countries that looked at the efficacy and safety of dapagliflozin 5 mg or 10 mg daily dose in T1DM inadequately controlled on insulin. After 24 weeks of treatment, significant and clinically important reductions were seen in HbA1c [mean difference from baseline to week 24 for dapagliflozin 5 mg vs. placebo was –0·42% (95% CI –0.56 to –0.28; p <0.0001)] and for dapagliflozin 10 mg versus placebo was –0.45% [–0.58 to –0·31; p <0.0001]), total insulin dose [mean difference in total daily insulin dose from baseline to week 24 was –8·8% (95% CI –12.6 to –4.9; p <0.0001) for dapagliflozin 5 mg vs. placebo and –13.2% (–16.8 to –9.4; p <0.0001) for dapagliflozin 10 mg vs. placebo] as well as body weight. There were no new safety signals and the drug was essentially well tolerated. The overall adverse event profile was similar to clinical study experience with dapagliflozin in patients with T2DM. Small increase in adjudicated definite DKA was seen with dapagliflozin which was manageable with standard care (1% each in the placebo and dapagliflozin 5 mg groups and 2% in the dapagliflozin 10 mg group). On similar lines, the DEPICT-2 Study, another phase 3 study evaluating the safety and efficacy of dapagliflozin 5mg and 10 mg doses in uncontrolled T1DM subjects over 24 weeks significantly decreased A1c (0.37% and 0.42% reductions in the DAPA 5 mg and 10 mg groups respectively), total daily insulin dose (TDD) and body weight versus placebo. As measured by masked continuous glucose monitoring (CGM), mean interstitial glucose, mean amplitude of glucose excursion (MAGE) and mean percent of readings within target glycemic range (>70–≤180 mg/dL) versus placebo (PBO) were improved. The results were same as in DEPICT-1 showing that dapagliflozin was well tolerated, improved glycemic control and decreased variability without increasing hypoglycemia but with more DKA events when used in uncontrolled T1DM patients as an adjunct to insulin. Both DEPICT-1 and DEPICT-2 went on to set the stage for use of SGLT-2 inhibitors as add-on adjunct therapy to insulin for adult T1DM patients uncontrolled on insulin who have a good understanding of the early warning signs of ketoacidosis, undertake regular home monitoring (including of blood ketones) and have a high level of self-monitoring and communication with their diabetes team. A 28-week extension phase of DEPICT-1 is in progress.

The North American inTandem1 Study evaluated the efficacy and safety of the dual SGLT-1 and SGLT-2 inhibitor sotagliflozin in combination with optimized insulin in patients with T1DM. This 52-week study demonstrated that sotagliflozin (200 mg dose as well as 400 mg dose) combined with optimized insulin therapy was associated with sustained HbA1c reduction [From a mean baseline of 7.57%, placebo-adjusted HbA1c reductions were 0.36% and 0.41% with sotagliflozin 200 and 400 mg, respectively, at 24 weeks and 0.25% and 0.31% at 52 weeks (all p <0.001)]. At 52 weeks, mean treatment differences between sotagliflozin 400 mg and placebo were –1.08 mmol/L for fasting plasma glucose, –4.32 kg for weight and –15.63% for bolus insulin dose and –11.87% for basal insulin dose (all p <0.001). Genital mycotic infections and diarrhea as seen more frequently with sotagliflozin. Adjudicated DKA occurred in 9 (3.4%) and 11 (4.2%) patients receiving sotagliflozin 200 and 400 mg, respectively and in 1 (0.4%) receiving placebo. Severe hypoglycemia episodes were fewer with sotagliflozin (6.5% patients from each sotagliflozin group and 9.7% patients receiving placebo). Patient-reported outcomes were improved with the drug while adjudicated

DKA events were slightly more in the sotagliflozin groups (3.4% and 4.2% with 200 mg and 400 mg doses respectively) versus only 0.4% in the placebo group.

A recent meta-analysis published by El Masri and colleagues looking at the use of SGLT-2 inhibitors in T1DM patients across four RCTs assessing canagliflozin, empagliflozin and sotagliflozin as add-ons to insulin and also dapagliflozin as add-on to liraglutide and insulin. The conclusion was very promising, showing not only the benefits of reduced insulin doses, weight and improved HbA1c in individuals with T1DM but also no significant increase in adverse events, hypoglycemia or diabetic ketoacidosis.

Though there is a lot of emerging evidence on the safety and efficacy of SGLT-2 inhibitors in T1DM patients, albeit based on short-term studies, the final word is yet awaited. There is a need for long-term studies establishing not only at the safety and efficacy but also similar cardiorenal pleiotropic benefits with these drugs in T1DM patients as have been seen in T2DM patients before these drugs can be recommended as novel add-on agents to insulin in T1DM patients with suboptimal glycemic control.

SAFETY CONCERNS

Most of the safety concerns with use of SGLT-2 inhibitors in T1DM are same as those in patients with T2DM. The incidence of GTIs and UTIs has been similar in magnitude and intensity as has been the reduced hypoglycemia rates as seen in studies of these agents in T1DM. There have been concerns on their long-term effects on bone health and increased fracture and amputation risk with these agents in patients with T2DM, hence it is pertinent to assess these effects in patients with T1DM who are already at higher risk for neuropathy, peripheral vascular disease, osteoporosis, fractures and amputations.

The slight increase in DKA events as in T2DM becomes a grave concern especially in the T1DM patients. The SGLT-2 inhibitors may increase the risk of DKA in these patients both directly as well as indirectly. The lowered glucose values may prompt these patients to inappropriately reduce their insulin doses to avoid hypoglycemia, exaggerating the insulinopenia. This insulinopenia may increase lipolysis, free fatty acid release and ketogenesis. Furthermore, these

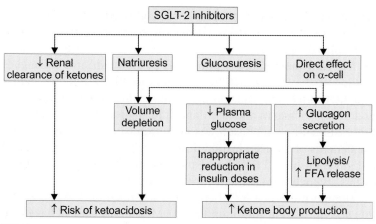

(FFA: free fatty acid).

FLOWCHART 1: Potential mechanism for sodium-glucose cotransporter-2 (SGLT-2) inhibitor associated increased risk of diabetic ketoacidosis.

drugs by lowering the renal threshold for glucose to almost 70 mg/dL may cause loss of large amounts of glucose in urine. Hence DKA may occur at mildly elevated glucose level, with the potential risk of delayed diagnosis of this serious condition.

Increased glucose loss may lead to compensatory increase in glucagon levels stimulating neoglucogenesis and FFA release. The consequently increased glucagon/insulin ratio further promotes ketogenesis. Furthermore, these agents by decreasing the renal clearance of ketone bodies with increase in plasma ketone levels may further delay the diagnosis of DKA. Most of the studies evaluating SGLT-2 inhibitors in T1DM as described earlier have shown a slightly increased DKA risk at even mildly elevated glucose levels as in T2DM, underlining the need for caution and regular monitoring for ketosis more so in patients with T1DM (Flowchart 1).

CONCLUSION

The SGLT-2 inhibitors today are recommended as novel agents with multiple pleiotropic benefits for patients with uncontrolled T2DM. Not only have they proved their safety and efficacy, but their cardiorenal benefits have established them firmly as preferred agents in all current hyperglycemia management algorithms globally for T2DM patients. As these agents work in an insulin independent manner, their role in T1DM has been a subject of much consideration, leading to multiple small, albeit short-term studies exploring their safety and efficacy as add-on agents to insulin in uncontrolled T1DM patients. All the emerging data seems very promising, calling for larger long-term studies that can establish them as recommended adjunctive therapy in T1DM. Recently, on the 4th of February 2019, the European Medicines Agency's CHMP regulatory committee has recommended AstraZeneca Forxiga (dapagliflozin) as the first oral agent that can be used as an adjunct to insulin in patients with T1DM with BMI above 27 kg/m^2 who are not having optimal glycemic control with insulin following promising results of the DEPICT studies. Regulators in Japan and the US are also reviewing the drug for use in T1DM, though it would be pertinent to wait till more long-term data can be generated.

SUGGESTED READING

1. Buse JB, Garg SK, Rosenstock J, et al. Sotagliflozin in Combination With Optimized Insulin Therapy in Adults With Type 1 Diabetes: The North American inTandem1 Study. Diabetes care. 2018;41(9):1970-80.
2. Dandona P, Kuhadiya ND, Ghanim H, et al. Adjunct Therapies in Type 1 Diabetes. Endocr Pract. 2016;22(2):277-80.
3. Dandona P, Mathieu C, Phillip M, et al. Efficacy and safety of dapagliflozin in patients with inadequately controlled type 1 diabetes (DEPICT-1): 24 week results from a multicentre, double-blind, phase 3, randomised controlled trial. Lancet Diabetes Endocrinol. 2017;5(11):864-76.
4. El Masri D, Ghosh S, Jaber LA. Safety and efficacy of sodium-glucose cotransporter 2 (SGLT2) inhibitors in type 1 diabetes: a systematic review and meta-analysis. Diabetes research and clinical practice. 2018;137:83-92.
5. Henry RR, Rosenstock J, Edelman S, et al. Exploring the potential of the SGLT2 inhibitor dapagliflozin in type 1 diabetes: a randomized, double-blind, placebo-controlled pilot study. Diabetes Care. 2015;38:412-19.
6. https://www.europeanpharmaceuticalreview.com/news/73381/ema-forxiga-type-1-diabetes/Feb 4, 2019.
7. Kuhadiya ND, Husam G, Jeanne H, et al. The combination of insulin, liraglutide and dapagliflozin astriple therapy for type 1 diabetes. Diabetes. 2015;64.
8. Mathieu C, Dandona P, Gillard P, et al. Efficacy and safety of dapagliflozin in patients with inadequately controlled type 1 diabetes (the DEPICT-2 study): 24-week results from a randomized controlled trial. Diabetes care. 2018;41(9):1938-46.

9. Mudaliar S, Armstrong DA, Mavian AA, et al. Remogliflozin etabonate, a selective inhibitor of the sodium-glucose transporter 2, improves serum glucose profiles in type 1 diabetes. Diabetes Care. 2012;35:2198-2200.
10. Pieber TR, Famulla S, Eilbracht J, et al. Empagliflozin as adjunct to insulin in patients with type 1 diabetes: a 4-week, randomized, placebo-controlled trial (EASE-1). Diabetes ObesMetab. 2015;17:928-35.
11. Yang Y, Pan H, Wang B, et al. Efficacy and Safety of SGLT2 Inhibitors in Patients with Type 1 Diabetes: A Meta-analysis of Randomized Controlled Trials. Chin Med Sci J. 2017;32(1):22-7.

SGLT-2 Inhibitors and the Kidney: Lessons Learnt from CREDENCE Trial

INTRODUCTION

Sodium-glucose cotransporter-2 (SGLT-2) Inhibitors have emerged as a revolutionary class of oral antihyperglycemic agents with a unique mechanism of action that goes beyond their designated purpose of glucose-lowering to reduce weight, regulate blood pressure and provide cardiorenal benefits as well. The three landmark cardiovascular outcome trials (CVOTs) namely EMPA-REG, CANVAS Program as well as DECLARE-TIMI have gone on to establish these agents as providing cardiovascular benefit by reducing both atherosclerotic events as well as hospitalizations from heart failure in a wide variety of patients. Owing to their renal mechanism of action, concerns have been raised on their use in patients with suboptimal renal function. Though all the three above mentioned CVOTs have gone on to demonstrate salutary renal benefits in improving renal outcomes, most of these agents have been recommended in patients with relatively preserved renal function at estimated glomerular filtration rate (eGFR) of 60 mL/min and above. The effects of these drugs on long-term eGFR point toward their potential role in mitigating loss of renal function through various plausible hemodynamic mechanisms. The Canagliflozin and Renal Endpoints in Diabetes with Established Nephropathy Clinical Evaluation (CREDENCE) Trial was carried out to assess the effects of canagliflozin 100mg daily on renal outcomes in type 2 diabetes mellitus (T2DM) patients with albuminuric chronic kidney disease (CKD) with eGFR varying between 30 and 90 mL/min/1.73m^2. The exceeding benefits lead to the data and safety monitoring committee recommending an early cessation of the trial after a planned interim analysis. The risk of kidney failure as well as cardiovascular events was demonstrated to be lower in patients with T2DM and kidney disease who were given Canagliflozin 100 mg daily versus the placebo, establishing the cardiorenal protective action of these agents in this population.

THE CREDENCE TRIAL

Methodology

This was a randomized, double-blind, placebo-controlled , multi-centric clinical trial that enrolled adult patients aged 30 years and above with a glycated hemoglobin level between 6.6% and 12.0% (6.5–10.5% in Germany due to their country amendment) with CKD, defined as an eGFR of 30–90 mL/min/1.73m^2 (calculated by the Chronic Kidney Disease Epidemiology Collaboration equation) and albuminuria (urinary albumin-to-creatinine ratio) >300–5,000 where albumin was measured in milligrams and creatinine in grams, as measured in a central laboratory. Almost 60% of the enrolled patients had an eGFR of 30 to <60 mL/min/1.73m^2 as per a prespecified plan. All these patients were on a stable dose of an angiotensin-converting enzyme inhibitor or an angiotensin receptor blocker for a minimum of 4 weeks before randomization. They were then prescreened for baseline eGFR and urinary albumin-to-creatinine ratio to meet the eligibility criteria and were then entered into a 2-week, single blind, placebo run-in period. Only the patients who had received at least 80% of single-blind placebo during the run-in period were then eligible for randomization.

The eligible patients were randomized in a double–blind 1:1 fashion to receive either canagliflozin 100 mg orally daily or the matching placebo using randomly permuted blocks, with stratification according to the eGFR category at screening (30 to <45 mL, 45 to <60 mL and 60 to <90 mL/min/1.73 m^2). During the trial, the CANVAS Program results were released raising a suspicion on increased risk of lower limb amputations. This lead to a protocol amendment in this ongoing trial in May 2016 mandating all investigators to examine patients' feet at each trial visit and temporarily discontinue the assigned treatment in any patient found to have an active condition predisposing to an amputation.

The trial was designed to be event-driven, enrolling at least 4,200 patients requiring 844 events to provide a 90% power to detect a risk of the primary outcome that was 20% lower in the canagliflozin arm versus placebo at an alpha level of 0.045 after adjustment for one interim analysis conducted by an independent data monitoring committee after the occurrence of the primary outcome in 405 patients. Detailed statistical methods used are outside the preview of this chapter and are available online in the detailed trial published in the New England Journal of Medicine.

Outcomes

Primary and Secondary Outcomes

The primary outcome was a composite of end stage renal disease (dialysis for at least 30 days, renal transplantation or an eGFR of <15 mL/min/1.73m^2 sustained for at least 30 days as per the central laboratory assessment), doubling of serum creatinine from baseline sustained for at least 30 days according to central laboratory assessment, or death due to renal or cardiovascular disease.

Secondary outcomes assessed in the study were planned for sequential hierarchical testing in the order as follows:

- A composite of cardiovascular death of hospitalization for heart failure; then
- A composite of cardiovascular death, myocardial infarction, or stroke; followed by
- Hospitalization for heart failure
- A composite of end-stage kidney disease, doubling of serum creatinine level or renal death
- Cardiovascular death; then
- Death from any cause; and finally
- A composite of cardiovascular death, myocardial infarction, stroke or hospitalization for heart failure or for unstable angina. All other efficacy outcomes were exploratory.

Safety Evaluations

In view of concerns raised about the different adverse events with this class of drugs as well as signals raised on increased risk of lower limb amputations and fractures seen with canagliflozin use in the

CANVAS trial, thorough safety evaluations including laboratory testing and assessment of all reported adverse events was carried out in this trial. Besides all cardiovascular and renal outcomes, key safety outcomes including fractures, pancreatitis, ketoacidosis and renal cell carcinoma were adjudicated by independent adjudication committees that were blinded to the trial-group assignments.

Results

Of the 12,900 patients screened from March 2014 to May 2017, a total 4,401 underwent randomization at 690 sites in 34 countries, with a similar match of baseline characteristics in both groups. The mean age was 63 years with a fair 33.9% representation of females. The mean glycated hemoglobin level at baseline was 8.3% and mean eGFR was 56.2 mL/min/1.73 m^2 along with a median urinary albumin-to-creatinine ratio of 927. Being an event-driven trial, the trial was stopped early once the requisite number of primary outcome events to trigger the interim analysis were accrued by July 2018, meeting the pre-specified efficacy criteria for early cessation. At trial conclusion after a median follow-up of 2.62 years, 27.3% patients in the two groups had discontinued therapy for different reasons, putting an adherence rate of 84% to the trial regimen during follow-up.

Effect on the Primary Outcome and Renal Components (Fig. 1)

The event rate of the primary composite outcome of end-stage kidney disease, doubling of serum creatinine level, or renal or cardiovascular death was significantly lower in the canagliflozin group than in the placebo group (43.2 and 61.2 per 1,000 patient-years, respectively), which resulted in a 30% lower relative risk [hazard ratio, 0.70; 95% confidence interval (CI), 0.59–0.82; p = 0.00001]. The effects were consistent across regions and other prespecified subgroups and for the components of end-stage kidney disease (hazard ratio, 0.68; 95% CI, 0.54–0.86; p = 0.002). The effects were also consistent across renal components, including the doubling of the serum creatinine level (hazard ratio, 0.60; 95% CI, 0.48–0.76; p <0.001) and the exploratory outcome of dialysis, kidney transplantation or renal death (hazard ratio, 0.72; 95% CI, 0.54–0.97).

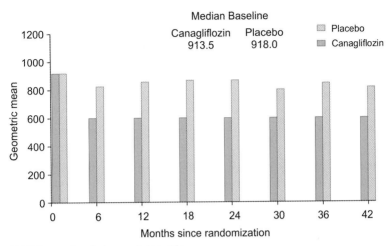

(A) Urinary albumin-to-creatinine ratio

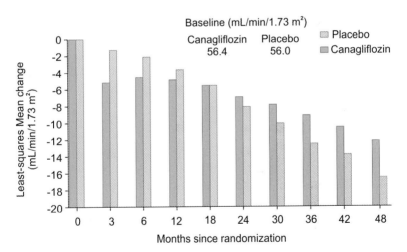

(B) Change from baseline in eGFR

Note: Panel A shows the effects of canagliflozin and placebo on the urinary albumin-to-creatinine ratio in the intention-to-treat population. Panel B shows the change from the screening level in the eGFR in the on-treatment population. The I bars indicate the 95% confidence interval in Panel A and the standard error in Panel B. The albumin-to-creatinine ratio was calculated with albumin measured in milligrams and creatinine measured in grams.

FIG. 1: Effects on albuminuria and estimated glomerular filtration rate (eGFR).

Secondary and Exploratory Outcomes

Lower risks of several secondary outcomes were seen in the canagliflozin group when tested in a hierarchical manner, including the composites of cardiovascular death or hospitalization with heart failure (hazard ratio, 0.69; 95% CI, 0.57–0.83; p <0.001), cardiovascular death, myocardial infarction or stroke (hazard ratio, 0.80; 95% CI, 0.67–0.95; p = 0.01), and hospitalization for heart failure (hazard ratio, 0.61; 95% CI, 0.47–0.80; p <0.001). The relative risk of the composite of end-stage kidney disease, doubling of the serum creatinine level, or renal death was lower by 34% in the Canagliflozin group (hazard ratio, 0.66; 95% CI, 0.53–0.81; p <0.001).

There was no significant between-group difference in the risk of cardiovascular death (hazard ratio, 0.78; 95% CI, 0.61–1.00; p = 0.05) so the differences in all subsequent outcomes in the hierarchical testing sequence were not formally tested as per the trial design. The hazard ratio for death from any cause was 0.83 (95% CI, 0.68–1.02) for the composite of cardiovascular death, myocardial infarction, stroke, or hospitalization for heart failure or unstable angina, the hazard ratio was 0.74 (95% CI, 0.63–0.86).

Effects on Safety Outcomes and Intermediate Outcomes

The rates of adverse events and serious adverse events were similar in both the groups with no significant differences observed in the risk of lower limb amputation as well as fractures in both the groups. As expected though rates of diabetic ketoacidosis were low, they were relatively more in canagliflozin group than the placebo.

The glycated hemoglobin level was lower in the canagliflozin group than placebo group with an overall mean difference of 0.25% (95% CI, 0.20–0.31). Similarly the canagliflozin group showed lower levels of systolic as well as diastolic blood pressure and body weight than the placebo group. The urinary albumin-to-creatinine ratio was lower by 31% during follow-up in the canagliflozin group (Fig. 1). The eGFR as expected showed a greater fall in the canagliflozin group in the first 3 weeks, following which the decline was slower in the canagliflozin group than the placebo group.

Interpretation

The above findings are very significant in establishing the safety as well as benefits of canagliflozin in type 2 diabetes patients with albuminuric kidney disease. The authors deduced that among 1,000 patients enrolled and treated with canagliflozin 100 mg daily in their trial for 2.5 years, the primary composite outcome of end-stage kidney disease, doubling of serum creatinine or renal or cardiovascular death would occur in 47 fewer patients in the Canagliflozin group than the placebo group (number needed to treat; NNT-22). Furthermore it was estimated that treatment with canagliflozin in these patients would prevent 22 hospitalizations for heart failure (NNT-46) and 25 composite events of cardiovascular death, myocardial infarction or stroke (NNT-40).

This goes on to establish canagliflozin as an efficacious treatment option for renal as well as cardiovascular protection in these type 2 diabetes patients with CKD. It is important to note that these benefits were observed over and above a background therapy of renin-angiotensin system blockade, the only known renoprotective drugs in patients with T2DM, putting things in a better perspective. While all the other CVOT trials included essentially patients with relatively normal renal function, CREDENCE comprised a population that was at a higher risk of renal failure and was designed to evaluate major renal end points as primary outcomes. Although the between-group differences in glycated hemoglobin levels, weight loss and blood pressure reductions were quite modest, patients in the canagliflozin arm fared much better in demonstrating an overall much lower risk of the primary outcome and lesser end-stage renal disease.

The concerns of potential harm with these agents due to an initial acute reduction in the eGFR were laid to rest suggesting that the benefits were observed independent of glucose levels and possibly attributed to a reduction in intraglomerular pressure besides other potential mechanisms under evaluation. Owing to the potential high cardiovascular risk of the trial population, it was heartening to see significantly lower rates of cardiovascular outcomes, including the composite of cardiovascular death, myocardial infarction or stroke in the canagliflozin arm. These findings were consistent with the findings of CANVAS trial with canagliflozin as well as EMPA-REG trial with empagliflozin and DECLARE TIMI 58 with dapagliflozin, establishing the cardio-renal benefits of this class of drugs in different populations.

The CREDENCE on the other hand further reinforces the renal safety and improved renal outcomes with canagliflozin in potentially high cardio-renal risk group of type 2 diabetes patients with albuminuric CKD. The overall safety profile of this drug also is consistent with the other CVOT findings, though the increased amputation risk signal in CANVAS was not seen in CREDENCE, the reason for which is still not clear, but may be potentially attributed to different trial population or protocols or could just be a chance finding.

To conclude, CREDENCE successfully demonstrates a lower risk of kidney failure and cardiovascular events in type 2 diabetes patients with albuminuria CKD with canagliflozin at a median 2.62 years follow-up establishing it as a potentially distinct agent for cardio-renal protection in such group of high risk patients.

Limitations

Though this was a well-designed trial, there are certain limitations one needs to be aware of. The early cessation of the trial at a planned interim analysis may have limited the power for some secondary outcomes and may potentially elevate the risk of overestimating effect sizes. However this is unlikely to majorly influence the findings observed in the trial as seen in the precise effects observed and their consistency with other larger SGLT-2 inhibitor trials. Furthermore, the off-treatment eGFR among patients who completed the trial was not measured, giving rise to maybe an underestimation in the differences in the eGFR values at trial cessation. Importantly, patients with advanced kidney disease, i.e. eGFR <30 mL/min/1.73 m^2, those with nonalbuminuric or micoralbuminuric disease as well as kidney pathology other than T2DM were all excluded from the trial, hence making it questionable whether these deductions can be generalized to such population groups.

SUGGESTED READING

1. Perkovic V, Jardine MJ, Neal B, et al. Canagliflozin and renal outcomes in type 2 diabetes and nephropathy. N Engl J Med. 2019. DOI: 10.1056/NEJMoa1811744.

Index

Page numbers followed by '*f*' indicate figures respectively.

H

Hazard ratio 24
Heart failure 65, 69
  development of 41
  hospitalization for 22
  prevention of 40
Hemoconcentration 56
  manifested 40
Hemodynamic 44
  effects 38-39
Hemoglobin A1c 3, 19, 23, 39,
  66, 69
Hepatic
  gluconeogenesis 8
  neoglucogenesis 53
Heterozygous FRG in benign
  condition 18
Hydroxyl functional group 4
Hyperglycemia
  chronic 1
  management of 13
  mild 35
  worsening 7
Hyperkalemia 73
Hypertension 21
  management, case for
    aggressive 35
Hypoglycemia 49
  risk of 72, 79
  agents 49

I

Immunoreactive insulin 39
Incretin axis 1
Infectious diseases, treatment
    option for 2
Inhibiting histone
    deacetylase 41
Inhibitory constant values 2
Insulin 4
  add-on to 66
  doses, careful titration of 79

resistance 65
secretion, improvements in 32
sensitivity 32
using triple combination
    therapy of 80
Insulinopenia 83
  degree of 53
Interstitial fibrosis 18
Intracellular sodium
  concentration 16
Intraglomerular hypertension
  in patients 46
Ipragliflozin 4, 26
  efficacy 60
Isoflavanoid
  glycosides 4
  based structures 4

J

Jaundice 4

K

Ketogenesis 46
Ketone 38
  body production,
    clinical significance of
    increased 34
  oxidation 41
Kidney disease 88
  chronic 65, 69, 87
  epidemiology collaboration
    equation 88
  failure, risk of 88
  progression 42
Kidney interstitium 16
Kidneys filter 17
Kurarinone 4

L

Lavandulyl functional 4
Leukorrhea 4
Lifestyle, management of 63
Lipids effects on 59

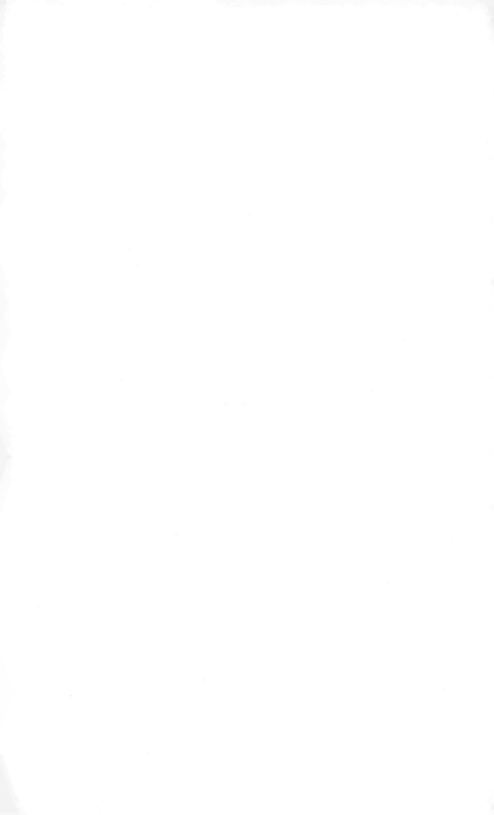